Dr. Gaffney's Coaching Guide
for
Better Parents and Stronger Kids

Carol Renaud Gaffney, Ph.D.

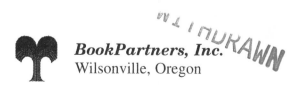
BookPartners, Inc.
Wilsonville, Oregon

BookPartners, Inc.
P.O. Box 922
Wilsonville, Oregon 97070

Dedication

To Chris, Sean and Kevin — you have taught me more about living and spirit than I ever thought possible. Each of you is a gift of light and love. As a young parent I hoped I would provide what you needed and wanted for your lives to be full. I had no idea how much I would learn from you. You are truly wonderful, and I thank each of you for your strength of spirit and purpose.

Acknowledgments

There are many people to thank for their ongoing love and support. I am truly blessed to have both my parents, Alphonse and Elizabeth Renaud, as continuing models of caring, persistence and the willingness to live each day fully. For over 25 years, Tom and I have been partners and parents in caring for our home and for our families. Together we have provided love, stability and numerous points of view on a multitude of issues. Together we have brought three infants to adults. Quite a challenge, quite an accomplishment!

I would also like to thank Dr. Paul Hardy for his friendship and his intelligent, insightful approach to understanding behavior. Dr. Chongbai Xia, in his dedication to healing, has taught me about peace and wisdom. Thorn and Ursula Bacon have had confidence in my "authoring," and for that I am truly grateful. Great thanks are given to Tiffani Stidham, who has been the backbone of the office. And, of course, I want to acknowledge the numerous mothers, fathers and children who have trusted me to be part of their families during their times of transition.

Table of Contents

Introduction

Times have changed!! It does not seem so long ago that parents could feel confident that providing structure, discipline and information was sufficient to keep their kids safe as they grew up. In a few short years parents have found they can no longer take for granted that presence and love alone are sufficient to ensure the safety of their children. Parents cannot take for granted that their kids will be attracted to mentors and other important people who will take them under their wing and help them develop safely. Of course, guidance, support and love have always been the parents' responsibility, but there has been a feeling of confidence and trust that "things will eventually turn out okay."

That times have changed and danger lurks in close places was seeping into my consciousness almost six years ago when the reality of our twenty-year-old son lying in an emergency room with skull damage, the victim of a vicious attack, made me open my eyes.

We received the Saturday morning call that Chris had been taken to the emergency room after being in a "fight" the night before. It turned out that the "fight" was a one-sided affair when two people emerged from the shadows of a building with shovels, ready to attack Chris and his three college buddies, who were on their way back to their apartments. Chris was the easiest target of the thugs and they struck him viciously on the side of his head. It was only good fortune that one of Chris's friends turned, saw Chris fall, and chased his assailant away before the raised shovel could give another blow.

The next several months were difficult as we waited through surgery and recovery, hoping and praying that when the healing was complete, Chris's function would be normal. Again, we were lucky. Chris has had no residual functional problem. But no matter how well his body healed, life and my beliefs about life have never been quite the same. An emotional wound remains. It is a daily reminder that the world I took for granted has somehow changed.

A change occurred deep within me. I can remember how angry I was and how, because there was no legal resolution (the assailants were never found), I had no place to direct my anger. I thought at first that if I could ever get my hands on the guys that did this to my son, I would rip them apart. With the passage of time, I decided that if I were able to confront them, anger and violence would henceforth be part of my being, not just in my life. I chose not to let that happen. I remember consciously making the decision to put whatever energy I had into Chris' healing, not into retribution. I decided to stand for something of value. I wanted this atrocious event to make a positive difference.

In 1990, I had been in the mental health field for several years, providing therapy for children, adults and families. When Chris was assaulted I became more determined to crystallize my thinking and techniques towards developing ways families can protect against violence happening to them. I realized there are two aspects to Chris's story: 1) He had put himself in a vulnerable position through a number of choices he made, and as a result he became a victim. 2) The perpetrators had come to a point in their lives in which their violent behavior, their contempt for human life, was an everyday choice. My goal in the book is to address the problem from both sides; to provide ways for our children to keep out of harm's way and to provide them with values and choices of behavior that will keep them from resorting to violence. The key to both sides is the parents, their awareness, their knowledge, their involvement in their children's lives and how they guide them to becoming healthy adults.

We raised our children in a relatively protected suburban environment. There were no gangs, and if illegal drugs were present, they were not apparent. Crime had not yet invaded our neighborhood; gunshots were not heard. We took a lot for granted. Although our children did not have the available corner lot that I had growing up, I didn't worry about their playing soccer, football and baseball games on the front lawn or going to the neighbor's house. We did not have an alarm system for our house or car and we slept with the windows open on the first floor.

Kids in high school got rowdy, got drunk at times, got into fights, especially on the weekend of the cross-town rivalry. This was not acceptable but not unexpected, as the same things happened when I was in school in the sixties.

We accepted the personal challenge to let the kids go and to let them grow. We let the natural consequences of their actions do the teaching, until the natural consequences got life-threatening. Of course, we were aware of drinking, driving, drugs, but these seemed to be under our kids' control and based on choices they made. We took the opportunity for input when we became aware of the presence of problems. However, except for awareness of injury through driving, which was so often the "other person's fault," our children were not taught to live defensively.

Our eyes were opened that day in 1990 with Chris's injury when random violence came into our lives and our vulnerability became all too apparent. Very quickly we learned that natural consequences now involved real danger and that the "other guy" had gotten out from behind the wheel of the car and was prowling the streets and alleys wielding shovels and, all too often, guns. The stakes had risen enormously. It seemed to happen overnight. As I became more aware of what kids were doing, I also became aware that the "problems" were not limited to "the other side of the tracks." Our neighborhood looks the same as it always has: well-kept homes, tidy yards, the sound of the lawn-mower whining on Saturday morning. Our neighbors are conscientious people who have their recycling bins out twice a week. But today our nice neighborhood has gangs, many of our neighbors have been robbed, junior high and high school kids go through metal detectors entering school, fights have become brawls with victims requiring plastic surgery. The teachers complain about the affluent, arrogant students who think life owes them. Many of the local kids don't "hang out" because there are too many guns. Drug addiction is a pervasive disease. The kids seem to be taking control in their world which is out of control. Violence and the effects of violence no longer happen to the other guy.

    Parenting in the nineties requires a more proactive approach. Times have changed. It used to be that social institutions provided for life's learning experiences and for teaching lessons. Now, in the absence of the social cohesiveness of the past, parents *must* take back the responsibility to coordinate their children's experiences. It is their responsibility to help make sense of what happens and to ensure that the experiences their kids are exposed to are the ones the parents want them to have.

    I am not so naive as to think that parents have total control over what their children experience. The control diminishes from the day children are born, and the children's perceptions of their experiences are never up to the parent. What I am recommending is that we parents increase the odds that children choose experiences that are good for them. Also, we must become "resource parents" to whom our children can come for love, understanding and wisdom when they have problems that must be solved. When bad things happen our children need us as a perspective that only experience and maturity can bring. This is the responsibility of the parents: to be the mature resource; the ones with experience who can help the child come to an understanding of what has happened.

    Parenting in the nineties requires fostering the development of independence and responsibility and balancing that with an appropriate level of guidance and limits. The goal as parents is to produce emotionally strong, healthy, independent adults. This can be done by providing our children with the environment that supports their social, physical, intellectual, emotional and spiritual development. To do this, parents themselves must be emotionally strong, healthy, independent adults. In the recent past years we have relied on others to care for our children: the schools to care for their intellect, the churches to care for their souls, the doctors to care for their bodies, the therapists to care for their emotions, and organized athletics to care for their physical development. It is time — it is imperative — that parents take back the responsibility to be the trainers, the coaches for all of these facets of their children's growth. The time is *now*. For stronger kids, we *must* be better parents. Providing the appropriate environment for your children is your responsibility. To this end, with the understanding that kids learn from our behaviors and our values, there are three basic principles:

1. You can take your kids only as far as you have been. They may progress beyond where you are in life, in learning and in personal standards and values, but if they do, it will be because of what they learn from others.

2. Raising children to adulthood is a gradual process of their learning and our letting go. Your decisions about how and whether you should intercede are based on the age and stage of the child at the time a problem is experienced. And further, once you decide how much of the problem you own as the adult, you solve your part of it then support your child in his or her problem solving.

3. Behavior, yours and your children's, is an expression of biology, psychology, social experience and the yearnings of the soul. The medical and behavioral health fields have been guided by the idea that behavior is a result of the interactions of our biology, psychology and social experiences. The time has come to take the next step and add the concept of the soul to the factors affecting the expression of behavior. The closer your behavior is to the expression of your soul's needs and desires, the more relaxed, confident and healthy you can be as an adult and your children can be during their childhood.

Part I

Know Yourself

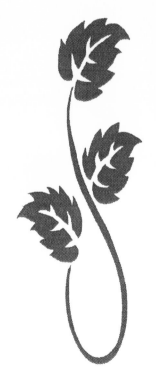

Know Yourself includes the information and exercises to guide you as you learn more about yourself. Know Yourself addresses the questions of who you are, where you are in life, what you want for yourself and what you want for your children. You will also be introduced to the steps that can help you have what you want. Know Yourself introduces simple, effective tools that you can use to make each day great. The materials are flexible and adapt to your uniqueness and circumstances. By the time you finish, your own personality and what you bring to your parent/child relationship will be evident. You will have a good idea of how you can be a better parent for stronger kids.

Chapter 1

You Can Take Your Kids Only As Far As You Have Been

This chapter about you, the parent, is first because "better parenting" is not about fixing the kids or making them behave. It is about you, your child and the relationship you have with him. Knowing each element of the relationship is essential to its working well. You would probably not go to a job interview without knowing about your strengths and limitations. Unfortunately, except under unusual circumstances, parents have been placed on the job without an interview, without a choice of children and without consideration of their job skills. Sometimes the match is made in heaven. But in any event, you must take the time to give attention to you, the foundation of the relationship. The stronger the foundation, the more stable the relationship will be when, inevitably, storms come through.

"You can take your kids only as far as you have been." Your children learn from you, not just from what you tell them, but from how you behave, which is a projection of your values and beliefs. Knowing yourself is the first step in helping you to assess whether you are the model you want your kids to learn from. It may also help you find something about yourself that may be provoking unacceptable behavior in your children. You will find that it is easier to change yourself than it is to make changes in someone else's behavior. You cannot do anything about your kids' genes, but you can certainly affect their environment. And part of their environment is you.

There is a growing understanding that trying to fix the kids without parental health and responsibility and input is just not working. Several communities and states are instituting parent responsibility laws. Recently a mother and father in a Detroit suburb were taken to court and found guilty of not exercising "reasonable control" over their 16-year-old son. The fine was $100 each and payment of court costs. This is not an excessive fine and probably will not be much of a deterrent, but the process may wake up a number of parents to what it is they need to do — that they cannot sit passively when their children become increasingly defiant and anarchistic. The point is that we as a society are saying "enough is enough" to kids who are out of control and the parents who spawned them. Some parents of teenagers are really adolescents (and younger) disguised as adults. Many of these parents share traits with their adolescents — they make a change only if there is a price to pay if they don't. This and other court cases may raise the motivation for parents to grow up and become actively involved in the parenting, coaching, guidance process with their kids.

There are many reasons some parents do not want to look at the part they play with their kids' behavior. One reason is that many parents are tired of taking all the blame for what goes wrong. Others are satisfied with who they are and don't find change necessary. Some parents believe that each person is responsible for his own behavior, therefore, any problems the kids may have are their own, regardless of their ages. Other parents think that they have already managed to change; it doesn't matter what they do; problems persist. Some parents are resistant to change because they think that if they change, they are admitting guilt or failure.

The majority of parents are more than willing to change, but they haven't been able to figure out why what they have learned to do still hasn't worked. Most parents are motivated, care about their kids and are willing to try something different. They read books, attend workshops and listen to tapes so they "know" what to do. But their knowledge and good intentions apparently disappear when they are home and faced with a real live "situation." The fireworks and confusion can begin much too quickly. Sometimes parents simply shut down; they simply can't do anything. Why can't these caring and well-intentioned people perform on the job? Often it is because of their own unfinished business. What does the behavior of Kathy staying in bed tell you about her parents? Are they exercising responsibility by allowing her to lie around?

"What am I going to do with Kathy? She won't get up in the morning. I go into her room three or four times and wake her up, and she ends up screaming at me to leave her alone. I can't stand it when she is mad at me." So her mother complains.

Kathy is nine years old and of at least average intelligence. She has no physical handicaps but does tend to be irritable and moody. Getting up on her own is a reasonable expectation for a nine-year-old. Getting cooperation to solve the problem would really help. If she does not want to cooperate with getting up, then it becomes the parents' work alone to let the natural consequences fall and act as the motivators. But parents are concerned that if they allow Kathy to get up on her own, she will be late for school and her grades will fall. At her age, Kathy should be accepting some of the responsibility for her grades and begin to realize that what she puts into it is what she will get out of it.

"But, I don't want to be late for work," the mother complains.

Good point — you do not want to punish yourself as you are solving the problems with the kids. Get cooperation if you can, because this is primarily Kathy's problem. But involve Kathy in the solution.

"Kathy, there's something that is going on that needs some attention. I don't think I'm going to be able to continue to try to wake you in the morning."

"Then how am I going to get up? You've got to wake me up; I can't do it by myself. I'll be late for school. I'll get zeroes. You can't do this to me. Don't you love me anymore?" (These are powerful controlling words, getting at parents on two important issues: academic performance and love. Guilt has just been invoked!)

"Kathy, those are concerns, and of course I love you. I don't know how you are going to get up. Do you have any suggestions? I've done what I can do. I'll be glad to listen to what you come up with. We can talk about it at the family meeting. Let's plan on this starting next Monday. What do you think of that?"

What stands between what you know and what you express is a filter made of your own hurtful experiences. It is the unfinished business of the past. This unfinished business comes up when you are in present situations that bear an emotional resemblance to past experiences. You may not know yourself well enough to wade through this "stuff" that is between what you want to do and what actually happens. You may think you are ready to say the right things to your kid, but when he has arrived home with terrible grades, unfinished homework, the chores half done, the dent in the car, the trouble with friends, the defiance of what you say, your words of choice become "choice" words. You are ready and willing to say the "right" words, but what comes out instead?

"I can't believe it's happening again!" (tears or shouts)

"When are you going to grow up?"

"You're just like your father/mother/brother!"

"I just don't know what I'm going to do." (crying)

"I can't handle this." (walking away)

You may cry or worry about what you may have done to make him like that. You may or may not empathize and understand that if the kid has "messed up" that badly, he probably feels worse than you do. (At least he should.) You may find that you become so upset and helpless that you lash out verbally and/or physically toward him. You may sit and cry and tell your child how much his behavior is hurting your feelings. You may leave, hoping that the problem will go away if you ignore it long enough.

If someone had been recording on video the last time you "had a problem" with one of your kids, what would the playback show? What would you hear? What would you see? What would you feel? Take a moment and visualize that encounter. Become the observer of what is happening. Examine the interaction in detail. Watch yourself carefully.

Now look and listen. What do you learn? What comes through along with the words and behavior? That's right: Emotion!! How does the emotion get transmitted? By "the voice" and "the face"; the "non-verbal" behind the words. Before you know it, the downward defensive or offensive spiral begins. Would you really expect anyone to be trusting with his feelings and forthcoming with information in that atmosphere?

"I would like to tell my mommy what I'm thinking, but I'm afraid of her. When I start to tell her and she gets mad, she starts looking like a witch to me. I know she's not. But she looks like one and I get scared and my mind goes blank."

"I feel too bad to tell my father what happened. He gets this hurt look on his face and I can't stand it. He already has so much on his mind and he is so stressed, I don't want to be more of a problem for him."

"I'm so mad at both of them, I don't really care what happens. They are so weak."

"I'm afraid to tell him anything, because as soon as I tell him something he doesn't like, he starts yelling. I can't stand it. He yells at everything."

How can this change? How can you clean that filter and manage your emotions, behaviors and family? How can you be the reasonable, calm, caring adult, the "life coach," when you are stressed-out, angry or depressed because of work, the messy house, the financial pressures, the lack of communication with your partner and the baggage of your own unresolved conflicts? Sometimes you have hardly a clue as to how to be a thinking adult rather than a grown person operating as a thirteen-year-old.

•••

These are some of the reasons to put effort into the Know Yourself questions on the next few pages.

The questions are about you, your child, and the relationship between you and your child. If you are not sure what a question means, answer in a way that is meaningful to you. Once you have completed the questions, take time to review your answers and your reactions.

I encourage you to put words to your answers by writing or speaking. I am sure you can think of many reasons for skipping this section or thinking that you know the answers or that just "thinking" the answers is sufficient. You are correct if you think that just thinking about the answers is better than skipping them altogether. But I can not emphasize strongly enough the difference that putting words to your thoughts can make. Writing is known to be effective in crystallizing ideas and as an aid to releasing emotions. If you don't want anyone to see your answers, write them on a separate piece of paper and then tear it up. If writing is not your thing, at least say the answers out loud, into a tape recorder perhaps. Somehow, get the answer out of you. Get involved in the process and the changes will occur more quickly.

Chapter 2

The "Know Yourself" Questions

A. *About you* :

1. Why are you reading this book?
2. What in your life provides the greatest satisfaction?
3. What is presently providing the least sense of accomplishment?
4. What are three adjectives others use to describe you?
5. What are three adjectives that you think best describe you?
6. Finish these sentences:
   I relax when _____.
   I get "uptight" when _____.
7. On a scale of 1 (not at all) to 5 (very much) you are:

Perfectionist	___	A problem solver	___
Moody	___	Responsible	___
Easy-going	___	Dictator	___
Anxious	___	A patsy	___
Excitable	___	Physically ill	___
Fun to be with	___	Stressed out	___
Controlling of others	___	Overprotective	___

8. How do your characteristics influence your parenting?
9. Who is someone you can talk honestly with?
10. What are you criticized for most often?
11. What do you criticize yourself for most often?
12. What are your "hot buttons"?
13. What are three sources of stress in your life?
14. How do you care for your "self"?
15. What is your life or soul's purpose?
16. On a separate piece of paper, draw a picture of yourself, using crayons. (No stick figures, please.)

B. About You and Your Kid :
1. With kids:
   What causes you the greatest problem?
   What causes the greatest joy?
2. Who has influenced your child-rearing/disciplinary techniques?
3. Why are you a parent?
4. What discipline patterns from your "family of origin" do you continue? (positive and negative)
5. How do your behaviors and attitudes affect the children you share your life with?
6. What is a strength in your relationship with your child?
7. What is one thing you can change which you think can make a difference in your relationship with your child?
8. On a separate piece of paper, draw a picture of you with your child. Again, use crayons, and no stick figures, please

Now that you have answered and reviewed the questions :
1. What question was hardest to answer?
2. What answer surprised you the most?
3. What do you know now that you didn't know when you started?

.

Chapter 3

Self-Care Versus Selfish

What was your answer to the question, "How do you care for yourself?" The answers I've heard indicate that self-care is not often considered by many parents.

"I think I put myself last on the list."

"I don't care for myself."

"I'm too busy to think about myself."

"I have to care for others before I can take care of myself."

"It's wrong to care for myself. That's selfish."

"Are you kidding?!"

These answers are profoundly important as they indicate the state of the caregiver. If you stop now, if you learn nothing more, consider your answer to the question, "How do you care for yourself?" Please believe that you must care for yourself and that it is not selfish to do so. In fact, self-caring is healthy and loving for you and for your family. Without evidence of your own self-care, how can your children learn to self-care from you? Without your ability to set personal limits, how can your children learn to set healthy personal limits for themselves?

Understanding the difference between self-care and being selfish is essential. You are being *selfish* when you do something for yourself while neglecting or ignoring the needs of others who have reason to rely on you for their well-being. You are *self-caring* when you do something for yourself in such a way that doing so does not compromise the well-being of someone for whom you have an appropriate responsibility. You have a responsibility to your children, but what you are truly responsible for changes as they grow older and have the competence to take care of themselves. You are totally responsible for them when they are infants when their needs must be put first. There will come a time when you no longer have to take care of their needs before you care for your own. In general, you are under no obligation to be taken advantage of financially, physically or verbally by anyone at any time.

The sooner you are aware of this, the sooner you will start eliminating negative influences in your life. Although this discussion is primarily about parents and children, the principles also extend to relatives, friends, co-workers and business associates.

It is easy to want to judge what someone else is doing, but attributing selfishness is difficult simply by observing another's behavior. For example:

Barbara is out shopping and is buying several new outfits. She has just had lunch with her friends and is arranging to play golf next weekend.

Randy has a new boat and spends weekends fishing with high school friends.

Sue is on a monthly shopping jaunt with her friends. Her three-year-old is staying with Grandma.

Bill has a number of committee meetings, has a trip scheduled to California next week, has several clients waiting to see him, and he is going out to dinner with a friend.

There is no way to tell from these scenarios who is being selfish and who is self-caring.

When we haven't been given permission to take care of ourselves, or if we think that it is selfish (and wrong) to do so, we can get ourselves into situations which are exhausting and discouraging. Are either of these two situations described below familiar to you?

Joe's children are in their twenties. He would like to retire, but the kids don't have steady jobs yet and they are living at home. He wakes up exhausted, wondering when it's going to be his turn in life.

Belinda is at her wits' end. She has cookies to bake, the house is a mess, she has just agreed to run the carpool, the baby is crying. She is exhausted but can't sleep. She looks in the mirror and can't believe what she sees.

Amazing things can happen when you understand what is reasonable and start asking for what you want. Take Mary, for example, who discovered that she didn't have enough time for herself because she was so burdened with household chores. When she heard that she wasn't being selfish to want more time for herself she asked for something she really wanted. Each person in the house would have to do his or her share of the housework. Now Mary has time to exercise or to read. How she uses the extra time is up to her. What really surprised Mary was that her husband had been willing all along to help. It was she who had assumed single-handed responsibility for the total burden, thinking that was what a good wife and mother should do.

When Joe asked his kids for help with the housework, they said they didn't have time. Joe decided they were old enough and physically able enough to manage by themselves. Because he didn't think he could enforce his decision on his own, he asked a friend to support him in his decision to ask the kids to leave. They finally did. They were not too happy about it, so they're not speaking to Joe. Joe is unhappy about his kids' response, but he has more energy, sleeps better, and is building a life for himself.

Obviously, selfishness versus self-caring is not a black or white issue. How you handle this is up to you, but if you look at what takes your energy, and find you are doing stuff that isn't yours to do, or you are being taken advantage of by people or things, put the brakes on and start saying "No." Determine what is right for you and what relates to your individual situation. Make decisions about your own behavior. What you do with your time involves balance and values which help determine your decisions. Examine your motives, understand your own "age and stage" and the responsibilities you have agreed to with others.

Saying "No" and being self-caring has become a lot easier with practice for me — it did not come naturally. I have had a very difficult time with self-care because I learned to believe that I should do for others before I did for myself. I think that's called being a "martyr." And, in addition, I became afraid to say "No" to people because I thought that if I did that would end the friendship. I am timid around disapproval, so there was a time when I said "Yes" to everything. I think that's called being a "wimp."

A number of years ago, I was baking cookies, serving on a lot of committees, telling my kids to hold on, wait a minute, because of other obligations. I remember one time when I was asked to do some cooking for a church function. I was pregnant, had two small children, my husband was working out of town, I was teaching piano and running the music program for the kindergarten. When I said, "I'm sorry, I can't" to a request for help, I heard the silence on the other end of the line. It was a risk for me to say "No," and the outcome was what I feared most. I soon realized it wasn't the end of the world and I had a great surge of strength realizing that my life was more my own than I had thought.

Although I've come a long way with most people, I still have some difficulty saying no to my children. This is because of my original belief that parents (and mothers especially) should always provide for their children if they can. This old tape still gets played at times, but when it does, I can more quickly turn it off. When it's off, replaced by the belief that parents (including mothers, which means me) provide what is needed for their children who do not have the capability to provide for themselves, I am more easily in "self-care." A belief such as this leaves me in the position of choosing what I am doing, rather than being obligated out of fear or guilt.

Chapter 4

All-Or-Nothing Thinking

The discussion of selfish versus self-caring brings up the notion of all-or-nothing (sometimes called black-or-white) thinking. Once you understand the limitations of all-or-nothing thinking you can free yourself to have numerous choices when "situations" occur. Having more choices leads to cooperation through less argument over who is right or wrong.

All-or-nothing thinking occurs when you believe there is only one way to do something in order for it to be "right" (which makes you good), and if you do it in any different way, then you are "wrong" (which makes you bad). When stuck with this belief, you limit yourself in trying new things. This can build up frustration and anger because you don't do what you want because of the fear of being "wrong." You will often find it necessary to justify your behavior to others and come up with a bunch of rationalizations for yourself. Also, if you think there is only one way to do something, you can start thinking of your kids as wrong, or bad, when they try something different. It just doesn't work that way. There are any number of choices that can be okay (neither good nor bad, right nor wrong). The determining factor for what you choose to do is ultimately based on your beliefs and the particular situation. Here are some examples:

Belief: Parents do everything they can for their kids:

"Will you do my laundry, Mom?"

"I'm sorry, I can't right now. Can you wait until tomorrow when I have more time?"

"I'm going out tonight."

"[Oh, dear. I guess what I want to do can wait.] Oh, all right, I'll do it now."

Belief: Parents do what they are reasonably responsible for:

"Dad, will you lend me your car?"

"I'm sorry I can't today."

"But you did last week."

"I know. I didn't have anything planned then, and today I've got something to do."

"Oh."

(Add a choice)

"But you know what, I won't need the car Saturday, so, you're welcome to borrow it then."

"Thanks, Dad."

Once you realize that each situation stands on its own merit, and you can make a decision based on today's circumstances and needs, you find yourself with numerous choices. I am not referring to being without standards and then deciding what works best for today. I am talking about choices that are made in reference to your beliefs and values which I am assuming are at least consistent with the social norms of your particular community. For example, I do not believe that children should be hit, so it doesn't matter what day it is, my choice would be something other than hitting. I value my body's health so I choose not to smoke. Also, I believe that I can decide how I want to spend my time and with whom I spend it. If you have beliefs different from mine, that does not make you "wrong" or "bad," it simply means we have differences in beliefs and values.

In fact, I can agree with something you say, which does not mean that I have to agree with everything you think or that I can't have an opinion that is different. I am also free to change my mind about something later. There is often such resistance to changing an opinion or agreeing with someone else that cooperation and real communication frequently cannot occur.

Have you noticed that some of the questions earlier in this chapter asked you to rate yourself on various qualities? I could have asked if you were anxious or not. Then you would have had to label yourself. Instead, I asked you to rate yourself. Instead of asking whether you are moody, I asked you to think about how moody you are, given that moods are normal human characteristics. And, it is not wrong or bad to have rated yourself in any particular way; it is a matter of understanding how those characteristics may enhance or interfere with what you want to do. The point is to give yourself a choice about what you do. If you want to do something for someone else, do it — just do it out of choice, not obligation. Do it not because you have labeled yourself a certain way because you think that makes you good. You are good, no question. Once you realize that, you can give yourself choices about what you do, including not being driven by a belief that leaves you feeling guilty or afraid to do something different. Consider this:

"Mom, will you do my laundry for me?"

"No, I can't today."

"But you did last week."

"I know I did, but that was last week and I didn't have this other stuff to do. I was able to do that for you when you asked, but this week, I can't. "

"Oh."

Real freedom is having the ability to choose what you want to do rather than being locked into responding to a belief system that may have been formed 20 or 30 or 50 years ago. That does not mean that you throw your values out; quite the contrary, just become aware of what you believe and see whether it fits for who you are today. One way of becoming more flexible is by becoming aware of each moment and responding to the needs or demands of that moment. Minding the moment and making the decision to do what the moment requires with a willingness to accept consequences constitutes freedom.

As you practice this form of decision-making, you can begin to build self-confidence. Self-confidence increases as fear of future failure diminishes. I want to be able to be on the path of choice, being able and willing to agree with another opinion or to be firm with an opinion of my own. At times I make decisions which are strictly for the well-being of another person and at other times I make decisions which are strictly for my own well-being. I don't want to be an all-or-nothing "in-the-box" thinker who is unwilling or unable to be flexible, or a person who does not understand the different options which are acceptable. For me, making a choice consistent with my values, appropriate to the situation with willingness to accept consequences constitutes personal integrity and freedom.

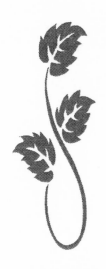

Chapter 5

Physical Illness And Stress

If you have frequent illness it is important to determine how much of this is due to being tired and stressed. Many people are surprised to learn that stress and illness can be related. Others admit having thought that stress was related to their illness, but have been afraid of being told that the "problem" was "all in their head."

Disconnecting physical illness from mental stress is a relatively new way of thinking. The "old" way (now regarded as the "new mind/body paradigm") of thinking about illness acknowledges the role stress plays in numerous physical and mental disorders such as hypertension, diabetes, fibromyalgia, migraine headaches, chronic pain, insomnia, ulcers, PMS, Raynaud's syndrome, depression, and chronic fatigue syndrome.

How do you know if you are under stress? Unless proven otherwise assume that you are! The question is to determine whether the stress you experience is positive and is enhancing your daily living, or whether it has become debilitating. Negative stress reactions can become additive and detrimental if there is not sufficient recovery time between stressful events. Even if there is no major trauma in your life you may experience numerous small stressors that accumulate. Even events that are positive and exciting are stressful because your system (body, mind and spirit) is required to adjust. Also, there is the personal consideration of how resilient you are to stress. This may be a family trait. Be honest. How much can you take before you start reacting (falling apart, zoning out or isolating yourself) or getting sick?

What is your environment like, and how does it affect your stress level? How much of a haven is your home? Is there a place for you to be private and quiet? Do music and television enhance your life or have you unwittingly allowed violence to enter?

I'm suggesting that you have lots of choices about your environment, and that the more attention you give to it and alter it to be pleasant, the more likely you and your family can be relaxed and healthy with each other. Science is catching up with folklore, and we have become increasingly aware of the impact of sights, scents and sounds on brain activity and, hence, stress.

What about your community? Do you experience your town or city as a community? How close are you to your neighbors? Are friends easily available? Is work a place of challenge and commitment? In small towns you may not experience as much environmental stress as someone living in a city with traffic, long lines wherever you go, air and noise pollution and increasing personal isolation and violation, but stressors are still there. What are you going to do? Most of you cannot and do not want to move. There are friends, family and jobs that keep you

....

where you are even if you know that some part of what goes on is not good for you. You find choices limited. You can leave; you can stay where you are and continue; you can stay where you are and make some personal changes. For most of us, staying where we are and making changes is the most reasonable solution.

I am willing to make some changes to adapt to my environment, and to incorporate activities to counteract the effects of the environment because I really do not expect the world or the people in it to change for me. It took me awhile to figure this out, but now that I am putting the effort into changing myself, I am making much more progress.

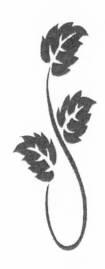

Chapter 6

Using The Breath

One change I made was to add moments and periods of intentional relaxation into every day. I had trouble finding time, as did most of the clients and parents I spoke with. Adding relaxation or self-care time for a nap or a bath or a walk or just time alone was too much to ask from a day that was already jammed. What I frequently heard was "I can't, I can't, I can't."

I became aware that Nature, in all her wisdom, has generously provided us with what we need to relax and to counteract the effects of the stress we experience. Nature has provided so we need to spend no extra time and no money to begin this process of relaxation.

What is it? It's been right under our noses all the time … the breath. Without it, we don't have much to worry about anyway, and with it, and with intention, we can begin the relaxation process which will allow us to begin the healing process. Just turning your attention to a single breath requires that you are in the moment, no longer worrying about what might happen tomorrow or next week, not regretting what you might have done yesterday.

You are built to take stress, and you are built to recover. There was a time when a person experienced stress and then had time to recover before the next big event. Because of the complexity of daily living in an industrialized society stress is ever present and when the stress does not let up, when you go from one situation to another without sufficient recovery time, the system eventually calls a halt through illness or reduced ability to concentrate, angry outbursts or burnout. Frequent experiences of the Fight/Flight Response (elevated blood pressure, heart rate, metabolism, breathing rate and muscle tension) interfere with the functioning of the immune system. This is serious! If you want, you can easily start building stress recovery times into your daily routines. With these recovery periods you can jump start the healing process. You can start counteracting the automatic stress response with intentional relaxation.

If you have any question about your health or wonder if breathing exercises will bother you, please check with your health care provider. If you feel uncomfortable at any time please discontinue the following exercise.

Begin by breathing as you usually do, noticing the breath as it enters your body and as it exits your body. Feel it come coolly in through your nostrils and leave with warmth over your lips or through your nose. Listen as it enters — and as it leaves. Notice where it goes: feel it enter your lungs and let your lungs expand. Feel it leave your lungs and let your lungs deflate — ahhhhhh.

With this simple action you have life. Your breath is simple and elegant. You were not taught to breathe, you cannot buy it at any store, yet, with your breath you have what you need for healthy, relaxed living.

How do you feel after this exercise?

Now find a comfortable position, either sitting up or lying down. Place a hand on your abdomen so your navel is covered. Breathe as you usually do. What happens to your hand? Does it rise, fall or not move as you breathe in? If it rises, then to some extent you are breathing abdominally or diaphramatically — a healthy, complete breath. If your hand falls, or does not move, as you breathe in, you are probably breathing with your chest muscles, which restricts the complete breathing process.

When you are ready, with a few easy steps and a bit of practice, you can breathe more completely and healthfully. It is easier for you to notice your breathing and to switch to abdominal breathing if you are lying on your back, but you can do this if you are sitting or standing. Again, place your hand on your abdomen covering the navel. If you are on your back, bend your knees. Breathe out first with a big sigh of relief or like you are blowing up a balloon. Then give a couple of "hoo's" when you think you are done with the outbreath. Like this — "hoo, hoo, hoo" — as you empty your lungs a bit more. Feel your hand going in, or falling. Now release your breath and as you breathe in your abdomen will rise as your lungs spontaneously fill with air.

When you are ready, take five complete, easy breaths. As you do this, direct your attention to your breath as it enters and leaves your body.

If you have been only half-breathing and have switched to full, complete breaths, you might feel light-headed as you get more air and oxygen. If you tend to be anxious, this could frighten you. Remind yourself that the dizziness results from the increase in oxygen. The more you intentionally practice this breathing, the more automatic the abdominal breathing will become, and the more you will be comfortable with the physical experience of relaxation.

Remember, when you are aware of your breathing you are in the moment. When in the moment you are truly experiencing your life. Sometimes we can become so involved with regretting the past or fretting about the future that we forget to be present in the only time we truly have — the moment.

With conscious breathing you can learn through experience the relaxing properties and the benefits of breathing deeply and completely. This intentional breathing can be used at will, anytime during the day as a mini-break or mini-relaxation. When is a good time? Well, anytime you need to relax or any time you think of it is a good time.

Go ahead and try it now. Breathe deeply into your lungs and be aware of the breath — the air entering your body. Breathe out fully, letting your abdomen drop as your lungs empty. Breathe in, allowing your abdomen to rise. Notice your chest filling from the bottom up until the top of your chest is expanded and full. Hold the breath at the top. Hold it as the wave holds for the moment before it returns to the sea. Then let your breath leave your body. Be aware of the emptying of your lungs, the sinking of your abdomen, the letting go of tension, the heaviness of your body.

Again, start with the breath entering and filling the bottom of your lungs first. Your abdomen rises. Your lungs fill from the bottom up and your chest expands. Continue for as many breaths as you like.

There are many ways of using the breath: a deep, one-time cleansing breath can work whenever you want it. Breathe out completely, almost pushing the breath out and getting as much out as possible. When you think you are completely done, push out, without straining, with three or four more breaths. Now let yourself inhale spontaneously, letting your lungs fill with clean air. Notice the sounds — the feelings — the smell — and the taste — of the breath.

As you are focusing on your breathing, you may find your mind wandering. A wandering mind is to be expected when you are stressed and beginning your relaxation. When you become aware of your wandering thoughts, acknowledge them and simply return your attention to your outbreath. Be easy and flexible with yourself.

There are many opportunities to use your breath for a mini-relaxation. You can simply direct your attention to your breathing while in the grocery line, the bank line or waiting at a red light. You can intentionally breathe while stalled in traffic or waiting for the kids to come home. You can now take advantage of this time to treat yourself rather than complaining about being stuck. You can breathe intentionally while sitting at your desk or while waiting on the phone or as a passenger in a car. You can direct your attention to your breath during a meeting or anytime that you need to relax. For those of you who are shy, no one ever has to know, unless you tell them.

Thinking clearly and making appropriate decisions about your behavior can be compromised because of perceived threats. When we perceive a threat the body responds to protect itself.

Breathing is so important because when you breathe intentionally and fully you start to reverse the effects of stressors that can trigger the Fight/Flight Response. Dr. Herbert Benson of Harvard University found the basis of eliciting what he called the Relaxation Response (decreased blood pressure, heart rate, metabolism, breathing rate and muscle tension) is a shift of attention away from disturbing events towards a chosen thought or activity, and using the breath. His research indicates that regular elicitation of the Relaxation Response has a significant positive effect in the treatment of many illnesses. In addition to better health, the better you are able to manage your breath and relaxation, the more options you are going to have as you manage yourself and your family.

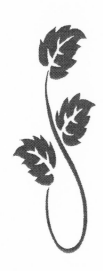

Chapter 7

Hot Buttons

How did you answer the question about your "hot buttons"? There is a nice formula that can help you to understand what your hot buttons are. I first learned of this when listening to "Chalk Talk on Alcoholism" by Father Joseph Martin. In his presentation, Father Martin refers to the formula, I over E except after D. When interpreted, the formula reads: Intellect over Emotion except after Drugs, implying that we generally are able to think before acting except after a trigger (in this case, drugs), when we operate on emotion (no active thinking going on.).

What are your triggers or hot buttons? What really turns you into an emotional wreck? I over E except after _____? Go ahead and fill in the blank. Is it one of your kids, a fall in the stock market, a bad day at work, an argument with a friend? I over E except after interacting with Johnny? After bad grades? After the kids fight?

If you have no idea, consider keeping a mood diary. It is simple enough: each time you "lose it," write down what happened, who you were with, and how you acted. As you look back on your "moods" after a few weeks, certain patterns will become evident.

I remember learning about one of my hot buttons from Leslie, a lovely eight-year-old who was having difficulty at school and at home. She was argumentative and oppositional and needed to be "right" regardless of the cost. I knew this, so I was prepared for her to try to get a reaction from me when we were together.

When I saw her one day she started:

"You're mean."

"You think I'm mean." (I am cool)

"You're the meanest person I know."

"I'm the meanest person you know." (I'm still cool because I expect some name-calling and I don't think I'm mean.)

"And you're old."

"And you think I'm old." (I'm warming up.)

"And you're an ugly, gray-haired, old grandmother."

My cool vanished and, although I kept silent, my face turned red, my eyes narrowed, and I thought, "How dare you say that to me." I was "gotten" and I learned what triggers one of my hot buttons — negative comments about my age and appearance.

It is important to know your hot buttons, whatever they are. When emotions control your responses, you are reacting, not responding. When you're stressed and you react, the old habits from your childhood surface. Frequently, that old stuff is what you heard when your parents were at the end of their ropes and couldn't cope. As you learn how you fill in the blank space in the hot button formula, your self-knowledge will be a powerful tool to maintain control. No one can steal your self-control — personal and internal — from you.

Chapter 8

Family Of Origin

I have heard comments such as:

"I'll never do what my parents have done."

"I've learned everything from them and now I do the opposite."

"I'm not a bit like my mother and father and if you think I am you don't know me or my parents very well."

"Enough is enough, parents have taken the blame too long. I am not going to blame my parents, and I don't want my kids to blame me."

"When you get down to it, I think my parents did a pretty good job, and if my kids turn out the way I did, that's not half bad."

Quite a range of responses! Even though you might have worked hard identifying and understanding your family patterns and are convinced that you will not make the same mistakes, there are times when your mouth opens and, as though a tape recorder was playing, words you heard as a kid pour out before you know it. What do you do then? Pressing the stop button on the tape recorder is usually easier said than done. When the tape is playing, you are running on automatic and there is no active thinking affecting your behavior. Returning to thoughtfulness and self-control is a necessary goal for reasonable interaction.

When you become familiar with your "family of origin" you may discover insights into your own behavior. Briefly, "family of origin" is a phrase that refers to the family that you grew up in, and more specifically how the family members and general environment affected information that now resides in your subconscious. This subconscious information drives your responses — thoughts, emotions and behavior. Your family of origin is where you inherited your genes, grew up and learned about how the world is supposed to work. Some of you might like to believe that you have nothing in common with your family of origin, but you do. You inherited genetic traits and you developed habits of responding from your family members even if they were not always present. You were influenced by the adults in your life in the same way that your children are now influenced by you.

You are a product of your genetics, psychology, social environment and spiritual nature. In order to understand who you are, and to make behavior changes, it is important to look at your family's traits: anxiety, depression, anger, alcoholism, violence, learning disabilities, attention deficit disorder, medical histories, personalities and personal histories including religious beliefs and values. You can start examining the patterns you inherited from the people in your life: biologically, psychologically, socially and spiritually. Your parents were your first teachers, but more immutable than what they said, or the actions that occurred, are the genetics and predispositions that you inherited.

Unless you have made intentional changes, the words and the rules you heard and saw as a child are now the voices that whisper inside your head and guide you as you make decisions. The early voices and rules have become values, attitudes and beliefs, and until they are examined and replaced, they will guide your decision-making on a subconscious level. These voices are made visible when you react in situations when you do not think deliberately, when you behave automatically. Fear, frustration, anger and excitement can push the buttons that start the old voices, and away you go. In the past you might have heard (and now hear yourself repeating):

"I can't believe you're doing this."

"When are you ever going to grow up?"

"Anyone with half a brain could do this right."

"You know better than to do this."

"What will people think?"

"I'll give you something to really cry about."

"How could you do this to me?"

The more angry and oppressive your own childhood experiences, the easier it is to be intimidating and mean around your own children. You may be aware that there are healthier ways to respond, but the accumulated and daily hassles (internal and external), better known as stress, sap the energy needed for a rational response. The result is that you react, rather than think.

Repeating certain patterns from the past has been very easy for me. Who do you think was standing next to a tan Suburban on the road to Santa Fe about eight years ago, pounding on an oversized kid? He was laughing, I was furious, as I pounded on him in the middle of the desert. So what did he do to deserve such a reaction? He was guilty of having too much fun in the back seat with his brothers, and not responding when I asked him to be quiet.

The tirades can go on and on and on. The kids have apparently tuned out, but their tape players are really pressed to "Record," gathering the information they will use with their own children many years from now. So much for enlightenment! Their thoughts? Similar to ours: "Mom, Dad, give it a rest."

An easy way to gain insight into your family of origin is to draw a family tree called a "genogram." On a large piece of paper, draw your family tree just as you would if you were doing a genealogy. Now, instead of just putting in dates of birth and death, describe family characteristics and secrets. What have you heard about Uncle Harry or Great Aunt Edna "going away for a while"? List the divorces, sexual abuse, psychiatric disorders, trouble with the law, physical abuse, abandonment, drug use, alcoholism, trouble with school, etc. Remember to include positive traits and accomplishments as well.

A note of caution: Investigating your family of origin is not an excuse for anger and blaming others for your problems; it is about learning more about the forces that shaped you — biological, psychological, social and spiritual. With that knowledge, you have real hope and an opportunity for change. Once you are aware of the unknown forces, you have a chance to live deliberately. When this subconscious aspect of life is first uncovered, many people are angry and feel distanced from their families. Your parents' lives were no more perfect than yours. Most of us had parents who were doing their best to fulfill their respon-sibilities. It is important to experience your anger, if it is there; but be careful how you express it — do not direct it towards another person. Of course, there are many of you who were neglected, ignored or downright abused, emotionally, physically and sexually. Addressing that reality is important so you can be free of the negative emotional connectors that permeate your family and your relationships with your children. Professional support and guidance is often helpful in negotiating that dark path. If you are angry or surprised, be aware of those feelings. But unless you know that someone intentionally wanted to hurt you, leave out the blame. No one is perfect, not even our own parents who we once needed to be perfect so we could feel safe. Now that we are big enough to take care of ourselves, we can start accepting and forgiving. Forgiveness releases a lot of energy that we can use to transform ourselves.

Knowledge about the family can also give you an opportunity to reinterpret your experiences:

"I was so surprised to learn that my father was having trouble at work and was depressed for most of the time I was in elementary school. My memories are that he would be cold and distant around me, that I couldn't please him anymore. I thought I had done something very wrong. Now I understand that he loved me, he just was not available because of something that was going on with him. So much of my anger with him and my lack of satisfaction with myself is dissipating."

"Family of origin" can be an extremely powerful influence in our present life. Understanding, forgiveness, and finishing the past frees up an incredible amount of energy that we can use to make today what we want it to be.

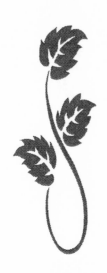

Chapter 9

Life's Purpose

The third premise is that each of us, including our children, has a unique soul. There are many definitions of soul and there are many names describing this nebulous concept such as self, higher self and spirit. For our purposes, they can be interchanged.

Who you are is an expression of your biology, psychology, social experience and the desires of your soul. The closer your life, the sum of your daily experiences, comes to expressing the desires of your soul, the more relaxed and happy and satisfied you will be. What does your soul desire? How close is your life to expressing your soul's needs?

As you reflect on these questions, look back at the picture you drew. What does it tell you about yourself? Are you happy, sad, angry, satisfied? If you are not happy or if you are unhappy with what you see in your picture, maybe there is a discrepancy between your daily life and what your soul desires. Dissatisfaction, annoyance and irritation are important emotional experiences, since they inform you that your behavior is inconsistent with a subconscious, deeper value or motive. What are your values and motives? If you are not doing what you want, why aren't you?

You may find these questions tedious if you think that it's impossible to fulfill your life's purpose because you are busy working at a job, keeping house, caring for your spouse, children and extended family. I hope that some of your "obligations" are also part of your understanding of your purpose. It is wonderful if your occupation is also fulfilling. If, as you review these questions, you find that your daily living does not satisfy on a spiritual or higher-self level, you may find yourself lethargic, frustrated, resentful or even angry. Your spirit's needs must be respected and behaviors consistent with them must be incorporated into your life for you to experience satisfaction from each day.

I now respect being present and living with purpose daily. Awareness of my own "life" purpose has taken time and cultivation. I also realize that my understanding of my purpose will continue to change as my additional experiences are integrated into daily living. I have become aware of my purpose when I have been quiet, when I remember what I have loved as a child, what provides a sense of joy and satisfaction. I have become aware of the necessity of "being," rather than being excited by how much I can "do." As a mother with three growing children I was aware of a purpose to provide nurturance, safety, love, opportunities for growth. As my children became older and more independent, I began to be more aware of the larger world I am part of. The incident in our family through Chris's experience reorganized my understanding of how interrelated we all are. We all share a connection to each other and what happens to one happens to all.

There are times when I am feeling content with who I am and how I am doing but the expression of the soul, once understood, does not show up automatically every day. I have to continue to be aware and stay focused. There is a struggle for me to be serene and calm as I am naturally "uptight," have been brought up to do the right thing (which often means that which others have done before me), and I tend to be reserved. This is a simple description of who I am, but the point is that in order for me to express my soul purpose, which requires that I present myself as well as information, I must respect these other aspects of me and do what I have to/want to anyway.

The first step in change is awareness. If you find spirit-based behaviors missing from your life, just be aware. As you continue in the next sections about self-evaluation and goal-setting, keep in mind how you can incorporate behaviors consistent with your soul into your daily routine. This is important for you to experience a sense of peace and wholeness.

As you become aware of your spirit, your individuality, the freedom and joy you experience as you live closer to your life's purpose, you will also understand how important it is for you to recognize this spirit within your children and to allow for its expression. A quiet child may not want to be a cheerleader or a football player. An energetic child may not find as much satisfaction from sitting quietly or reading or knitting as a more introspective child would. As you know yourself better, maybe even for the first time, and as you realize the importance of honoring your soul, you may become more empathetic to your child's need for acceptance of his spirit. Unconditional love for your children does not mean tolerating everything they do, it is about respecting and accepting their individuality even when who they are and what they want, is different from what you expected. Respecting their individuality and their accountability to the standards of behavior within the family are two separate issues.

Chapter 10

Living Intentionally

Now that you have a more objective assessment of who you are, your next step is learning to live with intention. The following section helps to evaluate your satisfaction with different aspects of your life. Once you evaluate where you are, you can then determine your priorities and start establishing goals in each of the areas as you begin the process toward balance and having the life you want.

Let each spoke on the illustrated Wheel of Life represent a rating scale for the area of life beside it. Translate '0' to mean not at all satisfied and '10' as completely satisfied. Now place a number from 0 to 10 on a place on the line that corresponds to the selected number. For example, if your satisfaction with health is a '3,' place the number 3 on the spoke to the right of the word "health." If your satisfaction with family is an '8,' place an '8' on the spoke to the right of the word "family." The '3' will be closer to the center and the '8' will be closer to the edge of the wheel. Continue in this way for each of the areas.

How satisfied are you with your health, family, and career? For those of you who have made a career choice of being at home, how satisfied are you with yourself in that role? How satisfied are you intellectually, spiritually, socially, financially? How satisfied are you physically, emotionally, and with your environment. (Remember, this is confidential, so go ahead and be honest.)

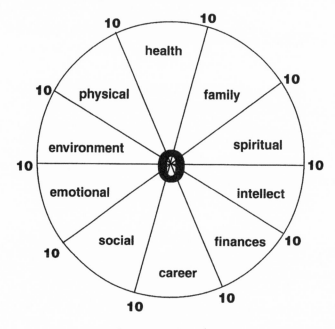

Wheel of Life

Now add the ratings you have made on each of the spokes and divide by 100. This number is your Quality of Life Index (QLI). This is your starting point as you progress towards a QLI of 1.0.

Once you have finished rating your satisfaction and have marked the numbers on the spokes, connect the

....

numbers to each other. This will inscribe a figure in the wheel. Because everyone is unique, the resulting figure will look different for each person completing the exercise. There is no right or wrong! This figure is not going to look like your mother's or your father's or your spouse's or your friend's. If anyone suggests that you should not have responded in a particular fashion, or shows surprise at the way you think, what are you going to say? Will you apologize? Will you change your answer?

Imagine that you are starting out on a trip in your car, but before you leave, you replace the right front tire with the figure that you have inscribed in your Wheel of Life. Imagine the kind of ride that lies ahead of you. Will it be nice and smooth? Slow? Bumpy? The shape of your tire will influence your ride, the one you have chosen. You may insist that you didn't choose your life up to this point. To a large extent this may be true, because many of your actions are determined by what you have been taught, so you really function on "automatic." Remember, if you don't have goals of your own, you will become part of someone else's goals. While that may be satisfying to some people, you must decide if it is satisfactory for you. As trite as this sounds, there is a relationship between the ride in your imaginary car and the ride you experience in life. If your wheel is asymmetrical, you may jolt, thump, and jostle down the road. If it is flat, you may never leave your driveway.

I remember a trip when our family was returning from New Mexico several years ago. It was about two in the morning as we reached the outskirts of a small town. With five people and ski gear from a week's adventure loaded into the car, we were anxious to get home. The ka-thunk, ka-thunk, ka-thunk woke me with a hazy understanding that something was wrong. One look at the flat tire was enough to tell us we couldn't drive further. We unloaded the car and pulled the spare tire out of the trunk. The good news was there was air in the tire. The bad news was that we had the small doughnut-type tire. We drove home cautiously, spending more time than we wanted. We arrived home drained, exhausted, and stressed.

Which category from the Wheel of Life is the most important for you to work on? What is the next most important area for you to address? Rank the areas in order of importance for you.

1. _____   6. _____
2. _____   7. _____
3. _____   8. _____
4. _____   9. _____
5. _____   10. _____

Are the categories listed with *your* priorities foremost, or did you hesitate and wonder what your (mother, father, kids, priest, rabbi, minister, boss, spouse) thinks of what you should list first? Did you check with the committee in your head to get permission before you committed to paper? Be honest. So many mothers believe they should be putting family as their first priority, when really what they want is to spend time developing another area that would help provide balance. How could they explain this to the children, spouse, their own parents? Many fathers list financial or career as their first priority because they think it's required, when really what they need for balance and personal peace is social or spiritual development.

As you get more involved in personal examination and goal-setting, share your goals and dreams only with people who will support you in reaching them. Being selective about sharing your dreams may go against early teaching because you've been taught that you are supposed to tell certain people (like your mother, father or spouse) everything. It is so difficult to come to a point of dreaming again and of having personal goals, that the last thing you need is someone criticizing you or telling you how you should go about accomplishing the goals. It is so difficult at times to follow through with changes in your life, that you owe it to yourself to choose people who will support who you are and what you want in life.

"I thought I knew what my priorities were until I actually wrote them down. Then they changed."

"I would have filled this out differently ten years ago."

"I understand that what I am writing down today describes where I am and what I want today. This can serve as a guide. It does not have to be written in stone."

"I've done this before, and I'm surprised to see how much progress I have made."

"I was surprised by my wife's response. She was jealous that I marked spiritual life first."

"What would they say if they really knew what I wanted?"

Are you satisfied with your priorities? Make your decision right for you, for today. The priorities and goals that you made ten years ago were right for you then. You are dynamic. You are changing. You are continually growing and learning. Yes, while you are parents and partners and responsible employees, your dreams and goals and needs and wants can change even as you continue in these roles.

It's when you forget about or ignore your dynamic nature that you wear out — body, mind and spirit.

Close your eyes, and take a long, full breath. Visualize yourself doing something that is important and pleasurable. The clearer and more detailed the picture, the easier it will be for this vision to become a reality.

Chapter 11

Goal-Setting

At this point, those of you who have been following the suggestions of this book will probably agree that writing or speaking your answers has helped clarify your thinking. Even though you thought you knew what you wanted, ideas have a way of crystallizing when they're expressed. Thinking, dreaming, prioritizing can be exciting, but the difference between a dream and reality can be in the process of joining words to your ideas. If you read business leadership and management books, you're familiar with goal-setting and written goals. Is it a bold idea to take techniques of business leaders and use these ideas as you guide yourself and your family to personal success?

Look back at your priorities and think about establishing goals in each of the areas from the Wheel of Life. Even though you have a top priority, you will find that some dreams and goals will overlap. For example, becoming involved in PTA may simultaneously satisfy needs for the family (doing something involving the children), social needs (making new friends), intellectual needs (working on a committee). A father may decide to include one of his children as he finds an activity that will benefit him physically and spiritually. A person who is active in all areas is more balanced and content.

Writing formal goals is a step up from having a to-do list, that daily list of important tasks. While writing goals is essential, there are ways to write your goals that can help increase the likelihood of their success.

Take a moment and write a goal for something in your number one priority area. Read what you wrote out loud. Now evaluate what you have written against the following criteria:

1. **Measurable** — Can you determine when the goal is reached? Can you measure it on a scale (such as weight, or number of times) or whether the goal is done or not done? (A hair cut is done or not, making your bed every day can be measured, being quiet when Karen comes home with a low grade, turning the television off after six o'clock; all are measurable goals.)

2. **Attainable** — Is this goal something that can be achieved or attained? Is it reasonable for you to think of losing fifty pounds in a week? Can you become the president of the company? Can you organize your paperwork in a day or a week? Can you reduce the number of hours you work from sixty to thirty?

3. **Personal** — Is this goal something that *you* want, or is this something that you are doing to make someone else happy? Do you really want to leave your job for more money or because your parents or spouse expect you to be a financial success? Is this goal consistent with your values and attitudes?

Also, does the goal involve behavior that you have

control over or are you thinking about controlling someone else's behavior? How can you force Johnny to go to sleep by eight o'clock? How can you make your kids get better grades? Having your daughter Rebecca attend Harvard may bring happiness into your life, but what about Rebecca's goals? Ask yourself whether you want your happiness to be dependent on someone else's behavior.

You can't force someone to do something he does not want to do without paying a price at some time. The only behavior you can control is your own, so set goals for what you can change about yourself. You can write a goal like asking someone to use a quiet voice when discussing bedtime.

4. **Specific** — Is this something you can visualize, is it tangible? For example, is the goal written in general terms such as, "I want to feel better"? You can't see "better"; you can't hold "better." You can visualize a smile on your face or laughing more. You can visualize eating healthier meals or cooking rice instead of french fries. Now you have something you can grasp, a picture of yourself taking action that will program your subconscious to make choices that are consistent with the goal. Using pictures, mental and real, is one of the strongest motivators to make a dream become reality. A picture is worth a thousand words. Advertisers use this concept daily. Put pictures to work to program yourself to achieve your goals.

To recap: When choosing goals, consider your soul; when writing goals consider the following criteria:

Measurable **A**ttainable **P**ersonal **S**pecific

The first letter of each word produces the acronym, MAPS. The goals you write will be the MAPS for your life journey.

Below is an example of a formally written goal. Please use this as a guide as you complete the empty sheet with a goal that represents your number one priority area.

Target Date: *7/31/00*
Areas: *Family Physical, Social*

GOAL — Measurable, Attainable, Personal, Specific (MAPS)
Spend two hours with the family having fun (meaning no purpose other than being together enjoying each other).

How is this consistent with who I am — Body, Mind and Spirit:
I want to be more present, available, connected to the people I love especially my children and spouse. I really want them to know me and I want to know them.

Steps to Achieving Goal — Target Date
1. Bring this up at a family meeting — 6/1/00
2. Block out the time on the calendar — 6/4/00
3. Write down inexpensive ways of doing things together — 6/1/00
4. When it seems easier to stay home and watch television or clean the house, be sure we do what we agreed to do. — 6/15/00

Possible Obstacles   **Solutions**

The kids might complain.   *Be firm about time together.*
No money.   *Find some activities that*
                                  are free.

•••

Target Date: _____
Areas: _____

GOAL — Measurable, Attainable, Personal, Specific (MAPS)

_____

_____

How is this consistent with who I am — Body, Mind and Spirit

_____

_____

_____

Steps to Achieving Goal — Target Date

1._____

_____ — _____

2._____

_____ — _____

3._____

_____ — _____

4._____

_____ — _____

5._____

_____ — _____

Possible Obstacles   **Solutions**

_____   _____

_____   _____

_____   _____

Now that you have at least one written goal, put it in a place where you can see it regularly. Keep the process of personal growth active. Enroll a friend you can trust, or hire a personal coach to keep you moving ahead. Inertia is a powerful force — use it to your benefit. You don't have to be in this alone, you just need to enlist people who accept you as you are, and are willing to support your dreams. You now have the knowledge and some of the tools to be a better parent. Keep at it — as you model energy and excitement and become all you can be, making each day great, your children can learn from you how to have dynamic, exciting lives.

Summary

That is it — all you ever needed to know about you — who you are, what you want for yourself. You now can write goals and you have an effective, no-cost tool for counteracting the effects of stress. Particularly, I hope you have a better idea of what your values are as they relate to your children. This information will guide you as you decide what is important and what interferes with your happiness and effectiveness as a parent. It is now time to understand who your children are, what they like and how you might best be with them.

Part II

Know Your Kids

The information in "Know Your Kids" is necessary for making decisions with and for each of your children. You have to know who they are, their strengths, their limitations, their likes, their dislikes, their temperaments and their desires. You must be aware of age-appropriate behavior and your children's maturity levels in order to decide how to coach them towards their own successes. As you develop clear pictures of each of your children, you can be aware of how each one's strengths contribute to a strong team effort within the family. To use a football analogy, Tom Landry never played Roger Staubach at defensive tackle. I am not a member of the local choir —

for good reason. There are many places that each of us can find a good fit for our talents and dispositions, so encourage your child to find his niche, then coach him to be as successful as he can be in his chosen position.

We make decisions about how to interact with our children based on understanding the Parent/Kid Triangles, which are displayed below.

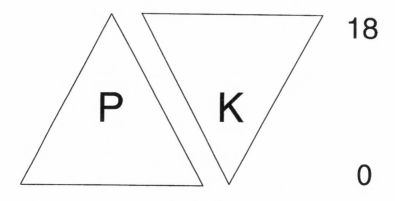

The "P" triangle represents the parents. The "K" triangle represents the kids. The numbers '0' and '18' on the right represent the child's age. The amount of responsibility each has is represented by the width of the triangle at a particular age. You can see that at age '0' a child has no responsibility for his well-being — parents have it all. They bear total responsibility for their child at his birth. Without the attention and care of an adult, an infant will perish. By the time a child reaches 18, the age in our culture when children traditionally graduate from high school, he needs to be completely able to make responsible choices. If you draw a line across the triangle at six years old and again at twelve years old, you can see how the responsibility for choices and problem-solving gradually shifts from the parent to the child. You can also see how the parent and child share in responsibility for solving problems. The intention to have children completely responsible for themselves by age eighteen is not because we are tired of being parents (although we may be), but because we know that unless they assume full responsibility for themselves when they leave home, our children can be vulnerable to harm, make poor choices, struggle on their own or eventually become dependent on someone else. Of course, being responsible also means knowing when to ask for help. An eighteen-year-old is not expected to have all the answers, any more than we expect to have all the answers. We want to raise our children to understand when to ask for help. We also want them to understand that asking for help is nothing to be ashamed of.

Please be aware that our relationships with our children do not end when they reach a critical age, it's just that our responsibilities for their choices and outcomes gradually diminish. As responsibility diminishes we can increasingly become a source of wisdom for our children.

Chapter 12

Raising Children To Adulthood Is A Gradual Process Of Their Learning And Our Letting Go

Growing up doesn't happen all at once! Physical, emotional, intellectual, spiritual and social growth all take time and experience. Luckily, our societies are set up with time to learn, and when this learning occurs gradually, stress is reduced for both kids and parents. The movie *Big* addressed this issue very nicely as Tom Hanks suddenly found himself in the adult world without benefit of time and experience.

You can compare the maturing experience to a homework project. I hear many parents say to their kids not to leave all the work to the last minute. "You'll never get it done," or "You just won't do as good a job." But, unlike homework, which can be completed early, maturity can't be done ahead of time — it has its own schedule. You can lay a great foundation for your children by providing many opportunities, but because genetics and experience are the important factors in maturing, well-rounded development is going to take the time that it takes, and time will not be hurried.

• •

Do any of these comments about children's maturity sound familiar?

"I can't wait until she's eighteen. Then she's on her own and I don't really care what she does then. All I want her to do until then is to follow my rules." (Mother of a fifteen-year-old)

"Kids know what's best for them. They learn by their mistakes, so let him go. His mother's too overprotective anyway. He's not going to get into trouble; this is what will make him a man." (Father of a seven-year-old)

"As I look back, I realize that in my attempt to have them learn on their own, I didn't provide enough good input. I wanted to respect their opinions and what they wanted so much that I ended up not respecting my own." (Mother of three adult children)

"I really wanted her to learn from my experience. I didn't want her to make the same mistakes I made. So I told her what she should do. I found out later that she resented every good idea I gave her because it seemed to her that if she did what I suggested, she would be doing it my way even though she had already thought to do it that way on her own." (Father of a twenty-year-old)

"I would die without my kids. I'm going to hold on as long as I can." (Mother of three young children)

Parents who are not black or white, all-or-nothing thinkers, will have an easier time with gradually letting go. If you do have trouble with flexibility, keep the Parent/Kid triangles in view as a reminder of the gradual process that growing to maturity is. The more you know about yourself and your child, the easier flexible thinking will become.

Maybe you hoped that your son Charlie was going to be a great football player or that Becky would be an accomplished ballerina, and maybe even though Charlie and Becky are talented in these areas, they have gifts and desires that push them in other directions. Mrs. Jones might be disappointed when she finds that her child, for whom she had aspirations from the moment of conception, is no longer growing in her image. As experience and research show, the more specific your expectations for your children, the more likely you'll be disappointed with what they become. Kids are smart enough to detect our subtle disappointments — and because they want to make us happy, they are often in the uncomfortable position of being unhappy regardless of what they do. When we can honor their wisdom to make their own choices, we can genuinely be proud and happy with those choices.

As the pictures of your children develop, I hope you also realize how their individual differences affect your relationship. It will become increasingly apparent that as similar as your children may seem, no two are alike and none of them is just like you. As much as you see yourself in them, they are not you. Each child has the right to have his individuality respected. Each child experiences the need for respect in the same way you have the right and feel the need for respect.

Sometimes the differences in each child are evident from the very beginning. As I think of the first months with my newborn babies, I can remember whether they fell asleep easily or were easily aroused. I remember their energy levels, their intensity, although they were tiny beings. I remember their responses to feedings, to having to have their diapers changed. What is amazing is that their temperaments as adults are similar to what they were as infants. There's often more acceptance for adults differing from each other, but be aware that the differences start from the first moments of life. All we have to do is notice!

A child's distinctive personality can cause problems for parents. Just when you think you have your parenting technique mastered, you find that what works one time loses effectiveness as your child develops and changes. Then you discover methods that work with one child are not necessarily going to work with another. Kids can certainly keep us alert. But once you know to expect the changes, the differences, you can be prepared to be flexible and to change with the times. Once your expectations are synchronized with reality, you can be prepared and can plan ahead.

"I didn't expect him to react the way he did. But when I stopped to think about it, Johnny has always been difficult when we've had to change plans. Next time I will think of what I can expect, rather than what I wish would happen."

"Mary is so grumpy when she gets home from school. I keep on hoping that she will grow up and get over it, but I guess what I need to realize is that when she is tired and hungry, and has been at school all day, she just is not fun to be around. Now that I realize that, maybe I won't expect her to be so cheerful and I won't be so disappointed."

While it's important to respect your children's choices, I am not referring to accepting antisocial behaviors, such as stealing, breaking traffic laws, using drugs or alcohol. Every society has limits, and you, as parents, are expected to establish these limits and to set personal standards within your homes. When the kids are living within these standards there are still many choices that can be freely made allowing for personal expression.

Chapter 13

Kids Are People, Too

Kids are people, and they have the right to be treated and valued as individuals. You may anticipate that your children will reach the magical age of eighteen, will leave home, find a job or go to college. This adult version of them may be one you can easily relate to — but our children are not merely miniature adults waiting to grow big. Neither are they shrunken adults or clones of us, an aunt or a grandparent merely waiting to carry on the family tradition. They are young humans experiencing the full range of human emotions, traveling through an incredibly important learning cycle that forms the basis of their personalities and values as adults.

Take a moment and remember a time when you were the age of one of your children. Let the memory become clear and focused. What do you see? What do you hear? What do you feel? Be aware of your mood, your temperament, your personality. As you experience this memory, become aware of how the people around you responded to your needs and feelings. Is this what you wanted or needed?

Could you express yourself? Were you told how to feel? Were you told that your feelings did not matter? Did you hear the phrase, "Children are to be seen and not heard?" Were you so busy pleasing the adults that you became unable to express your own feelings of fear or joy, sadness or excitement, hurt or pleasure? Were your parents so wrapped up in your success that you were unable to develop and separate from their needs for happiness? Were you afraid to tell important people about yourself because you might disappoint them?

When you were a child you dreamed. You hoped. Sometimes you were disappointed, scared or wanted attention, and sometimes you experienced joy and happiness. Your specific experiences have become your memories. Your children have the same fears, desires and dreams that you had as a child. Your children may not know how to express their feelings, but they do experience them. You may feel pain as you empathize with how they must feel at times. Once you acknowledge their feelings and give them permission to express them (not act them out) you are granting them freedom to be themselves. Rather than "stuffing" or ignoring their feelings because they don't want to make you mad or sad, your children can now start becoming comfortable with who they are and not be scared of what they feel.

"Don't tell me that — I can't stand to hear that you feel that way."

"How dare you feel that way. There is no need for you to be so upset."

"You shouldn't be so upset that your friend moved away; someone new is surely going to move in."

Compare that to:

"I'm sorry it's so hard for you."

"You are really upset, aren't you?"

Which would you rather hear?

Acknowledging that children are distinct people is an issue that I struggled with as my kids were growing up. It is embarrassing to admit how naive I was about knowing them as individuals. Even as an intelligent, educated person I had difficulty addressing this issue. Because of my own needs, wants and beliefs, I was often unaware of the effect my behaviors and choices had on their lives. At times I became overwhelmed with the demands of a busy life and family. Keeping house, getting meals and organizing finances were demanding. We had to eat, have a roof over our heads, and at times listening to my children ranked last on my list of activities. Spending time with them had to wait. They would be around tomorrow; the bills had to be paid today. I sometime avoided problems because I thought having problems were admission of failure for me.

I was naive, unaware, uninformed. Unfortunately, the apparent calm often meant I was ignoring the issues which brewed into storms later on. Once I realized what I was doing (or not doing) and that there were alternatives to avoiding or discounting my children's feelings, I was able to appreciate them more. This acknowledgment initially didn't make life easier for me. I realized that I could not make life easy (meaning without discomfort for them or me), but as I became more involved with what was really going on, life became richer; and the patina of smoothness was gone, replaced by a deeper, more stable rhythm.

I also recognize that, realistically, I could not have gone around second-guessing my every decision and making life perfect. The effects of my emotional trance were real. My lack of awareness became profoundly apparent when our family moved from the East Coast to Texas. Understandably, a decision to move is made by the adults; but our children were afforded little opportunity for input about how the move should proceed. Had we prepared them better, had we involved them in decisions along the way, (such as the process of packing and loading, deciding whether to fly or drive, how to manage the pets) the change could have been easier for everyone. I could have been so much more aware of their individual needs and responses, rather than treating our three children as "the kids" or "the boys." Our family would have been more of a team with common goals, each member doing his part to make the move a success.

Did the experience ruin them? No, of course not. Did it cause unnecessary distress? Unfortunately, yes. Had we included them more, they might have had more understanding and a sense of personal strength in the hectic upheaval of the move. Feeling strong and having some control are important in reducing the effects of potentially stressful experiences. Had they felt more control over their worlds, they might not have needed so much reassurance from us about what was going on. I took their demands and unruly behavior personally, instead of seeing that their needs for attention, reassurance and understanding, were certainly appropriate needs at the time.

If I had only realized that my turmoil was a symptom of my own uncertainties, I could have been more aware of the potential for difficulties for the kids. After all, I was the adult who had the capacity for insight and intentional change. Since they were so young, they did not have the language to express what was happening to them. A flower doesn't use words to say it needs attention, but we know that we must act when we spot wilting leaves. We take care to transplant a seedling, anticipating that it will need extra care and protection until the roots take hold. We need to be aware of signs from our children, just as we are with other living things. We often have been taught to rely on verbal language, forgetting the importance of the message in the behavior.

As our family made our transition, small things added up to make life difficult. We made a major move from a part of the country where our family grew up to one which was unknown. We left family and familiarity to begin an adventure in a new culture. I, as an adult, was generally aware of the changes to expect, but not prepared to deal with the specifics.

Several incidents during the first few months in Texas stand out in my memory. We moved in the late 1970s from a small New England town. When we got to our new home, we were graciously invited out to dinner. At the salad bar, I spied what looked like small pickles and piled them on. Such was my introduction to jalapeño peppers! The weather, even the sound of the wind, was different. Gardening in February wore me out. In 1979, there was only one miserly row of pasta in the biggest grocery store in town. I found that I was much more a creature of habit than I thought. I had to exercise before the sun came out. I found that my house got dirty quickly as I took advantage of every sunny day to spend time outdoors — it was always sunny in Texas. "God willing and the creek don't rise," took on new meaning after our first spring, with tornado and flood warnings every day for two months.

I was expecting, or at least hoping, that the children would jump in and adjust to this new life quickly. Had I stopped to think about the trouble I was having as an adult, I might have been more understanding of their adjustments. They were noticing differences from their former life; the way homework was assigned, how other kids dressed, routines at school which were new. Some teachers had as little experience with Yankees as we had with Texans. Each of these events meant an adjustment. I at least could ease slowly into the new community, but the two older boys were immediately plunged into school with many new kids and four new teachers in each grade to get accustomed to. Why did I want their adjustment to be quick? Adjustment meant I was doing things right and I certainly did not want to admit how helpless I felt. Also, I probably did not want to know how much distress the decision to move had caused them. Had the distress been acknowledged as normal and been dealt with, we would all have had an easier time. I wanted to ignore or deny the problems and just get on with it as quickly as possible. Don't problems just go away if they are ignored?

What I have learned is that when problems are acknowledged, when individuality is honored, kids can be cooperative and usually find reasonable solutions to problems. When they are acknowledged as people who feel things deeply, such as pain and joy, they feel real and accepted and not alone in their lives. When they trust us to be with them, they often trust us to guide them.

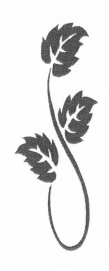

Chapter 14

Accountability

I have emphasized being sensitive to kids — who they are, what they need and how they feel. But, even when we are being "perfect" parents, the easiest children can be unreasonable and demanding. I do not think it is normal for children to be perfectly behaved. The question then becomes, how long are you supposed to tolerate unacceptable behavior? As kids grow up they must learn that life is not about having other people put up with them and their bad moods or testy, sarcastic comments. If they don't learn this they can become infected with the "center of the universe" disease.

When you are deciding how long you tolerate a particular behavior from your child, you can look back at the Parent/Kid triangle, check informational sources and figure out what is reasonable to expect. How old is the kid who seems so unreasonable? How much skill does this child have in self-control? How much self-control does he have? Is this child four, or ten or sixteen? Based on age and ability, can you reasonably expect this person to look at his own behavior objectively? If he can be objective, is he old enough and mature enough to start developing more acceptable ways of behaving? If so, that is when you can increase your expectations for accountability.

An infant is expected to have times of crying. A two-year-old can be expected to have temper tantrums. A thirteen-year-old can be moody and demanding. You can soothe an infant, a two-year-old can learn that temper tantrums are not acceptable, a thirteen-year-old can develop skills to be polite even when they don't want to be. *Even though behaviors are typical for an age, that does not mean that we give in to them;* it does mean that we set appropriate standards and levels of accountability at different ages.

As you can see, being sensitive to your child as an individual is different from his having to become accountable for his behavior. You may think that too much sensitivity to kids' needs is what has led to so much chaos in modern families. Nothing could be farther from the truth. Being understanding and expecting accountability are two different concepts. Accountability means that "house rules" are in place and are expected to be followed. Sensitivity means that your house rules are age-appropriate, within the kids' ability to observe and that when problems arise, you can be empathetic. In order to have accountability work, you need to understand your children's personalities and abilities so you don't fan a brush fire into an inferno. That means that with a two-year-old maybe you don't go to a restaurant which expects quiet behavior from you.

The chaos and rudeness so many kids exhibit is not because their needs have not been provided for. More problems have arisen from our giving in to our kids' demands and their notions of what they think they deserve.

....

Trouble also arises when we imagine we know what will make them happy or what we think they deserve instead of caring for their needs. What they *need* is really basic: food, shelter, love, affection, attention, opportunities to grow intellectually, opportunities to experience the consequences of their decisions, and time with their parents and families. Often what children want and think they need are material things that we also want them to have as tokens of how much we care for them. I have listened to many intelligent, angry teenagers complain that their clothing allowance is miserly, that their car is not new enough, that they're angry because their parents aren't giving them the newest and latest "stuff."

I want to reiterate that being an understanding adult does not mean accepting unreasonable behavior. Being understanding is a way of being with your child through his life. It is through understanding that a sense of unconditional love is developed. Demanding accountability for behavior is an expression of love even though children can get frustrated when they are not getting what they want.

Chapter 15

Letting Them Go, Letting Them Grow

Letting them go to let them grow is our motto throughout our children's lives. We eventually have to let go, so I advise that it be a gradual process rather than our holding on to them so tightly that they choke or that they fight so hard to get away, that we finally say, "I give up, you win. Live life the way you want."

Letting go is easier at some ages than others. The demands for independence also change with age. The demand for independence is stronger at preschool ages than it is during the elementary years. You know elementary kids are changing, but they don't announce it every day.

Adolescence is a time when the voice to let go thunders loud and strong. Adolescence is a transition time that is similar to the original birth. Before your child is born, his life and well-being are completely dependent on you. At a given point, hormones signal the end of this dependent phase. The message to the child is, "It's time to go on. It's time to become a separate person." During labor there is pushing and pulling, moving ahead and pulling back. With pain and perseverance, your child is born and required to breathe on his own.

The second birth occurs during adolescence when, once again, hormones signal the child. The message is nearly the same: "It's time to go on and separate more completely."As a parent, you know the time has come when the twinges of pain begin. The meaning of the pain may not be immediately obvious. It's usually only in retrospect that you realize when the metamorphosis began. This is another time of pushing and pulling, moving forward and pulling back. Just as with original labor, the experience of pain can be moderated by knowing what to expect and moving with the contractions, instead of fighting them. For both the parents and child, this is a time of anticipation and, perhaps, trepidation, since you don't know who will emerge when the process is complete. Actually, the fear of the outcome is shared both by the parents and child. The separation is made more difficult when anger, fear and resistance are involved. When this birth process is accomplished, your child stands on his own as an adult — financially, emotionally and physically independent from his parents. This individuation does not come just with age, it comes with experience and the support to be an adult.

I strongly encourage people to identify who they are and what makes them special and to take that information and fly with it. As parents, allow your hands to be open when your children want to fly off on their own strengths. The more you try to hold on to them, the more their spirits will be crushed since you will have to grasp tightly in order to keep them where you want them. When your hand remains open for them to leave, it also serves as a landing pad when they want to return.

The next pages contain a series of questions about your children. Again, as in the earlier exercise where you examined yourself, take the time to put words to your answers. Let the richness and diversity of the people you live with come into focus.

Chapter 16

The "Know Your Kid" Questions

(For simplicity, I will refer to your child as she. Make copies of the questions and complete one for each of your children.)

Child's name_____

1. How old was she at her last birthday? (Mark on the triangle.)
2. How old is she emotionally? (Mark on the triangle.)
3. How old is she intellectually? (Mark on the triangle.)

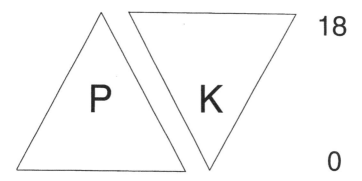

....

4. What are her assets?
5. What are her limitations?
6. What are three adjectives that describe her?
7. What are her hot buttons?
8. What skills does she have to handle the problems she encounters?
9. On a scale of 1 (not at all) to 5 (very much). How much is she:

Perfectionist	_____	Problem-solver	_____
Moody	_____	Responsible	_____
Easy-going	_____	Dictator	_____
Anxious	_____	Patsy	_____
Excitable	_____	Physically ill	_____
Fun to be with	_____	Stressed out	_____

10. What, if any, problems with health and development has she had?
11. How has this affected her?
12. What about her pleases you the most?
13. What about her irritates you the most?
14. What is her best tactic for getting what she wants?
15. On a scale from 1 (poor) to 5 (great) indicate how good her relationship is with:
    Dad   _____
    Mom   _____
    Brothers and sisters   1. _____
                                       2. _____
                                       3. _____
15. If you could change one thing about her, what would it be?
16. What do you most often disagree about? Agree about?
17. What do you want in life for her?

18. What do you think she wants for herself?

Are your expectations consistent with what she wants for herself?

Based on what you believe is reasonable for her age (check with the resources if necessary), how satisfied are you with her development in the following areas. As you did for yourself, mark along each spoke with:

0 = not satisfied at all, and ranging to 10 = completely satisfied.

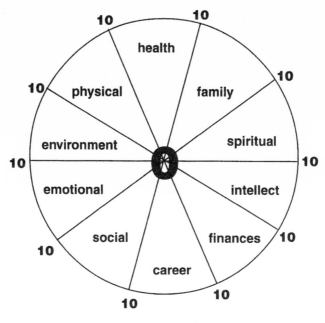

Wheel Of Life

Add the numbers on the spokes and divide by 100 for her Quality of Life Index. QLI = ___.

Based on the information that you now have, what do you need to be aware of as you interact with your child?

What answer surprised you the most?
What have you learned?

Chapter 17

Reasonable Expectations

What is reasonable to expect from children as they mature? Is development going to be easy and steady? No, it's not. Are kids going to continue to grow and change? Yes, they are. Will some periods be easier than others? Yes, certainly. Will you be annoyed or resentful at times because their schedule for change does not match your plan for your life? Yes, you probably will. Is it all worth it in the end? I hope you find it to be. You will have to wait to find out, but if you can worry less about the outcome and concentrate on what needs to be done today, you will have a better chance for overall satisfaction as a parent. Having kids and raising them is not a project that is going to be graded when you are done. It is an ongoing, day-to-day experience, in which you can find satisfaction even in the unexpected ups and downs. Today is all you really have, you don't have to wait until life is over to decide its worth.

Children grow and change at predictable but uneven rates. The process of growth and change is predictable. Children will walk before they can run. They will read words before they read sentences. They will learn to play with one friend before they learn to play in groups. They will learn to count before they learn to add. Hormones become influential before you see the physical indicators of change. These changes are predictable. It is predictable that our children must mature socially, physically, emotionally and intellectually in order to be fully functioning adults.

The rate of change for each of these systems and the schedule for these changes are different for each person, based on genetics and opportunities for learning. The changes are predictable, but timing and duration for each person are not. The schedule of change is unique for each child.

The more you prepare yourself for the changes and learn to identify the cues that indicate a change is taking place or is about to take place, the more in control of yourself you can be. The more you know about the person who is changing, the easier it is to make choices about coaching that person to success.

The majority of parents I counsel lament that they had no training to become parents and that kids do not come equipped with a manual. (They did not come with a warranty or a money-back guarantee either.) You can't buy a small appliance without an instruction manual these days. For kids, you have to rely on your innate knowledge or well-informed friends, or you have to go find a manual. Where do you get information about the expected changes? My "Baby Bible" since the early seventies has been the *Child's Development Series* put out by the Gesell Institute. This is my "manual" for learning what to expect at each age from birth through adolescence.

Many parents have called me in a panic wondering

about an attitude change, new fears, changes in diet, complaints about parents or friends. This is similar to developing a new rattle in a familiar car. Once the "manual" is checked for age and developmental expectations, many parents breathe a big sigh of relief as they realize that most of these changes are normal.

When you know what is reasonable for each age, you can begin to separate the normal from the problematic behavior. Sometimes normal and problem behaviors look a lot alike! A quick check in the "manual" can relieve a lot of pressure and anxiety as you realize that wildly fluctuating moods, "out-of-bounds" behavior, "I love you, I hate you" are sometimes signs of normal change, not an indication that your child is headed for the local detention center.

Remember: children are going to grow at predictable but uneven rates, and it is reasonable to expect variations in development. They keep changing! Physical, emotional, social and intellectual changes occur simultaneously. Does this sound too complicated? Well, becoming an adult is complex. But you do not have to have a degree in child development to be a good parent. I have met lots of people who have read lots of books and are only marginally effective parents. Then there are other parents who have not read any child-rearing books but who are naturally sensitive and empathetic and know when to say "yes," when to say "no," and when to say, "I'll think about it and let you know." Having the manual and this information is not going to make you perfect. There is no more humbling job than being a parent!

Chapter 18

Limit Testing

Among the predictable changes in a child's lifetime is that he go through patterns of testing limits. No parents have reported to me that their child thanked them for establishing a bedtime, mealtimes, study time, curfew, chores or expectation of good manners. Only as adults may we thank our parents in retrospect if they provided expectations and/or limits for us. If you remember that you did not thank your parents until *you* were an adult, perhaps you can be patient about getting thanks from your own children. If you need frequent "thank you for being a great parent" fixes from your kids, please get over it. Being an adult parent requires delayed gratification.

Limit testing is normal and there are messages associated with it. One message is: "Hey, Mom and Dad, I'm ready to try something new. I'm ready to go on. I want to be more responsible for myself. Please allow me the chance to move ahead."

Another reason for limit-testing is because children want an answer to the question: Are there limits? A "yes" answer lets the child know he is safe with the adults in his life and that he can settle down with confidence to learn the tasks of his particular age. Because children often do not know what questions to ask, the only way for them to get the answer to their question is to run a quality assurance test, using behavior.

What looks like limit testing can also be a cry for help due to unhappiness, depression or discouragement. Discerning the motive for behavior usually provides more of a clue to what is going on than listening to their words. The key is being sensitive to what is normal for your child and what is normal for the age so you can make a wise decision on how to proceed. Unfortunately, there is not a "magic formula" for how to make decisions. Judgment calls are involved. The more experience you have, the more informed your decision about how to proceed.

Do you have to tolerate the limit testing? Life would be so much easier without the hassle. Dealing with limit testing can be a huge energy drain. But don't be so quick to complain. For those of you who have established limits, at least you know that if there is limit testing going on, you have provided limits in the first place. For those of you who have not established firm limits and expectations for your children, please consider starting soon. If you institute limits when the kids are older, expect trouble. It is much easier to loosen the belt than to pull in the reins.

Limits are *essential* for healthy development. Limits provide the basis for developing self-discipline and delay of gratification. If you are concerned about the limit testing — if you think that it is too often, too forceful, or uncomfortable in some way — you can evaluate whether the limits you set are reasonable. If you find that your limits are not reasonable for the age and stage of the child, re-evaluate and change as necessary. If your limits and standards are reasonable, carry on, but listen more closely to understand the message that your child is sending.

As with understanding your child's individuality, being a sensitive, caring parent does not mean that you tolerate obnoxious behavior. Knowing that offensive, difficult behavior is normal for some ages only provides information on what to expect, but not what to allow. Accountability is still necessary. The lessons children learn when they modify unacceptable behavior are essential for development. These lessons include tolerating frustration, delaying gratification, coping with disappointment and learning cooperation. As children mature into adults, they must learn that they are a *part* of a universe, *not* the center of it.

I believe strongly in the need for limits and structure for safe development. In my work I meet families where there are no limits or the limits in place are not sufficient to protect children during vulnerable, impressionable times. Because our children know so much more about the world than we did at their age, we might mistakenly believe they also have the maturity to cope with this fast-paced environment. They can learn information at almost any age; however, understanding it and interpreting it takes maturity. Most children are exposed prematurely to violence, fear and trauma, and often in the homes where they need to find safety. I am not referring only to violence between family members, but from the music children listen to, movies and television news that show graphic events that I, for one, prefer to avoid. It doesn't make sense for parents to work hard to provide safe neighborhoods and then allow shootings, stabbings, trauma, blood and gore into their homes via the media. Why not provide age-appropriate protection for children? Does this seem overprotective or unrealistic? I'd rather err on the side of caution. I believe that children rely on us to keep them from danger until they have the skills, mentally and physically, to separate fantasy from reality and to take care of themselves. Until they feel safe, they can not complete age-appropriate development, and, as a result, delay the process of becoming emotionally mature adults.

Review the Parent/Kid Triangle for a reminder that growth to adulthood is a *gradual* process with behavioral expectations based on the age and developmental stage of the child. You make decisions about what is reasonable behavior and how to interact with them based on their ages. The other part of that is that each age and each stage has certain tasks to master before children can effectively work out the demands of the next stage. For instance, in school we have to obtain a passing grade before we move on to the next math level. Unfortunately, in life you can't go back to an earlier age, because life keeps pressing on.

When kids have no limits or the limits are not sufficient and appropriate to their ages, they become untrusting and fearful and learn they must take care of themselves. They often start taking on roles they are not mature enough to handle. As humans, we must take care of survival needs first. Kids are smart and do what they have to do to survive. However, the danger is that when they are focused on taking care of basic survival, it's difficult for them to develop socially or intellectually.

Kids will test limits to find out how safe they are. When they are not safe, they are intuitively aware of it.

Thus, it's essential for adults to set limits and provide order in the world. Once you set limits, what you can reasonably expect is that kids will challenge them, because that's exactly what kids are supposed to do. When they are testing limits, you can breathe a sigh of relief about how normal they are.

Chapter 19

Kids Who Can't And
Kids Who Won't

If your expectations are reasonable and your child's problems continue, you can evaluate whether your child is able to respond or whether or not he is intentionally acting out. Dr. Foster Cline distinguishes between kids with problems as "kids who can't" and "kids who won't.'

A "kid who can't" is one who, for some reason or other, is limited in accomplishing age-appropriate tasks. The limitations can be physical, intellectual, emotional or social. Do lethargy on the one hand, and overexuberance on the other, interfere with success? Could the problems stem from an undiagnosed illness such as diabetes, attention deficit disorder, hyperactivity, or allergies? Is your child tearful or unwilling to participate in age-normal behaviors because of depression or anxiety? Does your child have difficulty completing homework tasks because of intellectual or emotional limitations? Is this child moody or usually happy-go-lucky? Does he have difficulty getting along with other children? Are these problems caused by a lack of experience?

Any of these problem — depression, anxiety, physical limitation (including those not visible to the eye), attention deficits, poor vision, hyperactivity, intellectual limits, learning differences, moodiness, unpredictability, social delays — may influence children's behavior. These kids are considered "kids who can't."

The "kids who won't" are oppositional, argumentative, and try to win at someone else's expense. They are often mean and aggressive. Some have a history of "bad" behavior and seem like con men or women in the making.

Many "kids who can't" become "kids who won't" after a pattern of discouragement and continued failure, when self-esteem plummets and anger sets in. They often worry about what's wrong with them, or become discouraged and angry about their lack of success no matter what they do or how hard they try.

One question can often help you determine what type of kid you are dealing with. Simply ask him whether or not he wants to make the changes you have in mind.

"Bobby, we are really concerned about your low grades. Before we start putting any major effort into this we want to know if you are as concerned as we are. We want to know if you want to make some changes."

If the answer is "yes," you can move ahead and coach this kid to make the necessary changes. This will require time and support from the parent. Changes do not usually happen overnight, but at least you know you are playing on the same team.

What if the answer is, "No, I'm not concerned. You just expect too much. My grades are fine the way they are." Or, "I don't know." Or, "Who cares?" Answers like these often draw the parents' wrath because deep down the parents know that if the kid doesn't want the same things as the parents, there is little likelihood of achievement in this area. Parents have some choices now. These might include upping the stakes (bribery, which is a short-term fix and will backfire in the end), deciding whether or not to pursue the change, or continuing to pursue a conversation that might result in a change of thinking with this kid.

Developing a good relationship with a kid who does not want to try is very difficult. Getting around control battles is an extremely important strategy because, typically, these kids will do anything to win. Opening up dialogue, being aware of feelings, addressing the feelings rather than the behavior are helpful tools to remember. Patience is important, but because kids who don't want to try are so exhausting, being patient is difficult. Professional help is usually necessary. Groups such as "Tough Love" are good support systems for many parents who are struggling with this type of relationship with their children.

When you are making a decision on how concerned to be and what to do about a particular behavior, consider the total package that your child presents rather than picking on one particular troublesome attribute and then throwing your negative or angry energy at that. If your male child has long hair and earrings but has reasonable grades, is respectful to you and of house rules, and helps around the house, you can respond differently than if he is bringing home failing grades, frequently breaks house rules, has poor conduct at school, and generally exhibits lack of cooperation. Anger is not going to help anyway, so use your good judgment and use your energy to coalesce the relationship rather than picking your kid apart, piece by piece.

....

What do you do with the "kids who can't?" Getting a professional evaluation is recommended for determining what they "can't" do. If your child can't read because he is far-sighted, then corrective lenses are usually prescribed. If your child is diagnosed with ADHD (Attention Deficit and Hyperactivity Disorder), medication along with family counseling on how to structure the environment is often recommended. If there is a medical problem such as diabetes, medical attention is essential. It is important to realize that once the corrective measures have been implemented, the child is expected to be accountable for behavior, at home, at school and in his community, based on his age and new capabilities.

Parents often feel guilty if it turns out that their child has inherited a "problem" from them. When parents feel guilty or sorry for their kids, they can handicap them by not expecting them to meet the family standards. When guilt is motivating them, parents can easily make excuses for their kids' choices. It is not a limitation that becomes the disability, it is the parental attitude that the standards for behavior have changed and the child is no longer held to the family standard of acceptable behavior.

Of course, you can be empathetic with your child's feelings of sadness or embarrassment or feeling "less than" when problems are identified. But empathy does not mean you take on their feelings or change your standards or feel sorry for them. You may feel sad, but that is different from feeling "sorry for." Pity often has us interfering in parts of problems that are not ours to solve. Feeling sorry for a child will not help, but empathizing with feelings of loss or sadness can make him feel more understood and loved, which provides the basis for personal strength.

Your pity for your child may come from your own unresolved issues about yourself. You realize how much you suffered from certain problems and the last thing you want is for your kids to suffer as you have. You can spend your time agonizing over why the problem had to happen, or you can use the time to come to terms with the issue and move ahead. Here are two different ways of handling common situations.

"Everyone in my family is fat. I hated being called names when I was a kid. It made me miserable. I'm still miserable about it. When he [my son] started getting fat I knew it was going to be the same thing all over again. I've been so miserable ever since I realized that he is following right in my footsteps."

"She came home and said she had no friends at school because she had thick glasses. My first thought was that I knew this would happen, no one liked me and now no one likes her. I could have cried. Then I realized that wearing glasses has nothing to do with who you are or whether you are worthy of being loved. I didn't come to that understanding until I was an adult, so I decided to hold off on the lecture. Instead, I just listened to her pain. Before I knew it, she was finished and went out and played."

Summary

What about those kids! I hope you now have a deeper appreciation for the young people who live with you, who depend on you, who love you. Now that you better understand your children and what to expect from them, it's time to move on to learn the strategies that will help you have the relationships you want.

Part III

Know The Ropes

Know the Ropes includes information to use with your kids so you can be effective as well as caring parents. There are no tricks, there are no secrets, just basic skills — skills you can learn and skills you can use. A word of caution — regardless of how "good" you are, regardless of what you change, there is no guarantee that your children will "turn out" the way you want. In fact, the more specific your dreams for what they should be doing, the more likely you will be disappointed in what they choose. As you let go of making them become what you want, you may even enjoy being with your kids more. Remember that each of us has a spirit, a soul, a purpose. As parents we provide the opportunity for the child's healthy physical and emotional growth so their spirit can thrive. As you experience more success yourself, confidence and effectiveness will increase when you're dealing with your children.

Chapter 20

Reminders

As you develop new skills you may get discouraged if you or your kids do not make the expected changes as quickly as you would like. Remember that change takes time!

1. Take time to plan how you approach your goals. Use the goal sheets from Chapter Eleven to state your goals clearly and to develop the steps to reaching your goals. At the very least, write down what you want to change on your daily to-do list.

2. Change one behavior at a time. Trying to change too much at once leads to overload, frustration and failure. When being a parent gets too tough, it is easy to become discouraged and fear that the changes are not going to work. Focus on one change and when you are satisfied with your progress, move on

3. Start with something where you can guarantee success. Nothing breeds success like success! It does not matter if the one thing you change is as simple as smiling when you come in the door after a day of work. Whatever you try, however small, a change that works is a step in the right direction.

4. Real change takes time. Early efforts seem to reap large rewards, then the rate of change diminishes with time. In other words, there is more change in the beginning — just like being on a diet. Be patient. The even line of a learning curve is actually an average of successes and failures. If you could examine the reality of a learning curve, you would find many peaks and valleys.

5. An object at rest likes to stay at rest. Your kids are invested in life staying the same even if they are miserable. There is a certain comfort in the status quo. When you start making changes that affect your children you will probably experience resistance from them.

The message: Plan, keep it simple and be patient. There are a number of opinions about how long it takes for a new behavior to become a habit. Some experts claim that if you do something for thirty consecutive days it will be a new habit. According to others, in order to change a behavior it takes a month of the new behavior for every year a habit has been in place.

So, if your child is irresponsible about his belongings and is five years old, it may take five months for the changes you want to become a routine. (Also, keep in mind what is reasonable for a five year-old.) When I first heard this I was quite discouraged because I was going to have to wait more than a year for the changes I wanted from my oldest son. Then I realized that the month for every year ratio also applied to my changing my parenting habits. Once I accepted this sad news I realized that I had been learning to parent from the day I was born — not the day that my first child was born. I was discouraged at the thought of waiting more than three years to effect the changes that I wanted immediately.

When I was learning "new" ways of behaving as a parent, at times, I responded automatically with the old, critical, angry comments. As soon as I realized what I was doing wrong, I would stop, start again, and correct my behavior. The kids would sometimes do a "double take," but I was determined to replace the healthier responses for the old, automatic ones. I knew that the more opportunities I had to say it "right," the quicker my new behavior would become habit. One day, when a low chemistry grade was presented, I started with the usual litany of, "If you hadn't watched Monday Night Football and studied instead, you probably would have done better. If you …;" at which point I heard myself, stopped, breathed, thought and then said, "I want to start over. I'm sorry about that grade. I hope it works out better next time. If you want to talk about it, let me know."

I had the most difficulty with being mindful of the "new" ways when I was tired and otherwise stressed. I was pretty critical of myself when I kept making "mistakes." As I became more patient with myself and didn't expect perfection, I became more patient, less critical and accepting of the kids. The same critical voice that lashed out at my children was the same one I had carried chattering in my own head, castigating myself. This insight came suddenly, but not quickly. It came after methodically working on changing my behavior. The effort not only made day-to-day problem solving easier, but has paid off because I now have wonderful relationships with each of my children.

If you are not getting the results you hoped for, rather

than giving up, give yourself time to figure out what's going wrong. It's easy to think that these "techniques" work for "the other guy." Have patience; otherwise you might think the hoped-for changes are not worth your time or effort.

Be creative and try out a number of alternatives until you get the desired effect with *what feels right for you.*

Keep evaluating your plan. Go back to *Know Yourself,* review the information and check to see if there is something you have overlooked or forgotten to consider. What behaviors are interfering with the success you want?

Parents are sometimes afraid to be firm with their children, so they tolerate unacceptable behavior, grades, language and rudeness. Are you afraid that your child won't like you anymore if you are firm and Johnnie or Suzie does not get his or her way? Are you afraid of the conflict that might occur? Are you afraid someone might criticize you for trying something new instead of doing what has always been done in your family?

Do you have the energy to follow through or are you so involved with work, committees, or finances that you have little left over for parenting? Is the plan to implement change well developed? Are your expectations reasonable? Have you given your plan enough time?

If you are on your own in making these changes, you may want to enlist the help of a friend, family member or personal coach to help you stay focused and moving ahead. Don't be afraid to ask for help, but be sure whoever you ask is really on your side.

Changes can be made if both parents are not working together, but they may take more time and your kids might take advantage of what they perceive as a chink in the parents' armor. Kids have a wonderful way of sensing the

....

weak points in a relationship and working to divide and conquer in order to get their way.

A more serious problem develops if one parent is not only unsupportive, but actively interfering with the strategy you've laid out. This problem is between the adults and the adults must be careful not to vent their frustration and anger through the children. Parents in this situation are advised to carefully evaluate their relationship and tend to their problems.

Now check through your *Know the Kids* responses to determine if you missed or failed to consider an aspect of your child's personality. Does your kid not respond like other children? Does your child want to cooperate? Does your child understand that a change is expected? Is the desired change something he is capable of? What is the quality of your relationship with this child? How well do you communicate, or does the conversation consist of lectures and orders? The skills provided here will work with most kids most of the time; they may not work with "kids who won't." If you have a question about whether your child wants to cooperate, ask him. If he answers "no," at least you know where you stand.

Change adds stress to a family. Both you, the parent who planned the change, and your children, who may not agree that a change is necessary, will also feel the stress. The effects of the stress can show up in behavior that gets worse before it gets better. You may hear accusations like, "You don't love me anymore," or "I don't love you." These are powerful words to a parent, and indicate that you're being pressured through guilt to change your mind. Also, when you start implementing changes you may behave like a human pendulum — as far as you have been to one side of center, you can swing to the other. So if you have been a seriously lenient parent with few boundaries or rules, you may seem like an ogre to your kids when you begin setting limits, even though you know they are reasonable. Another problem that occurs is that children often become confused and feel abandoned when you no longer solve their problems, but instead encourage them to find their own solutions. You can try to explain that you love them enough to give them the chance to learn responsibility, but it probably will not mean much to them at first.

Whatever *you* are feeling, assume that your child is also experiencing some of those feelings, but without the intellectual or emotional maturity to understand or articulate his experience. Because of the lack of emotional maturity and the sense of helplessness that often accompanies youth, feelings may be magnified. Kids often rely on behavior rather than words to let you know they are unhappy. Be understanding, but maintain your course. For example, going to the pediatrician and having your children immunized may be painful for them, but you are not going to forgo the treatment because you value the long-term benefits. Discipline and setting limits may be uncomfortable for both of you initially, but it is the right thing to do as part of a plan that has an eye to the future.

You may think at times that you are swimming upstream. Becoming a better parent often means that you are setting standards (and sticking with them) that you think are right even though 99 percent of the families in your neighborhood are doing it differently. Sticking with your standards is very difficult if social experiences are jeopardized and your child is angry with you and claiming he feels like a nerd. If you are saying "no," make certain your reason comes from your values, not because you are having a bad day or you are angry with your kid or you don't want them to have a good time because your childhood was so bad. If you believe that you have established your priorities and values, are persisting with an intentional, planned change and have left your anger and resentment behind, be patient. But just get started — the sooner you begin, the sooner you will have what you want.

Chapter 21

The Basic Principles

There are four basic principles of healthy family management to keep in mind:

1. Sidestep control battles.
2. The person who "owns" the problem is the one best suited to solve it.
3. House rules should be clearly stated and, preferably, written down.
4. Family meetings are essential for smooth family operations.

1. Sidestep control battles

There is no reason to go to war with your own child. One way to avoid war is not to engage in needless skirmishes. You often hear about avoiding control battles, but I prefer the notion of sidestepping them. Sidestepping implies that these issues are addressed at another time, not simply forgotten or ignored. The same problems will continue to come up until they are intentionally addressed.

By sidestepping control battles, you say or act only in

a way necessary at that moment to stay consistent with the house rules. When new situations occur, parents maintain the right to say "no" without explanation at the time the event is occurring in order to think about what to do. In general, as parents, you only take the power or control you need and let your child take care of the rest. Stay available as a coach when your children are trying something new. Even though we learn from our mistakes we also develop skill and confidence from success. It is important that we are supportive with our children and not set them up for failure. Then you can support your children in their problem solving if they ask for help. All of us, including our kids, need control over some part of our lives. When you only exercise control over a part of a problem, your kids will learn that they have a say in what is going on. When they get to decide what they are going to do, they can be much more agreeable.

Sometimes we have to step in and make decisions not only about what we are going to do but what the kids are going to do as well. In this case, if you are not able to sidestep or avoid a control battle, if a decision about a conflict has to be made immediately, engage carefully so that you can be sure to win with dignity and not damage your child's self-esteem or self-confidence.

Sidestepping does not mean giving in, although it may appear that way at times. It is not giving in because there are consequences for unacceptable behavior, and ongoing problems will be addressed later. Even though giving in does not seem to make sense, it is what happens when parents try to save the relationship and their own dignity or are just too tired to fight. Giving in or giving up is not what you want your kids to expect from you. When you give in, kids think that you are a pushover or patsy and that they can intimidate or out-talk you. They learn they can get what they want if they just push long and hard enough. They may also begin to question how safe they are with you. But, you can postpone addressing a hot issue when you have confidence that you are going to address it at the next family meeting or when emotions are cooler. You can forgo an immediate battle for later conversation and negotiation. This way of handling an issue is not giving in, it is being reasonable.

You do not want your kids to learn that they can control you by "driving you over the edge" or into behaving in an embarrassing or shameful way. Once you think you "owe them" or have to make up to them because of how poorly you behaved, guilt and fear influence your responses. When you operate out of guilt, you lose your confidence to do what you think is right. Instead, you can become drained of energy and exhausted, and kids will take advantage of your weakened state to get their way.

Unfortunately, there are times when control battles are inevitable. You must realize this fact in order to be ready to respond. When you are prepared to respond, when you have a plan for emergencies, you can maintain your dignity by being calm and firm rather than threatening and angry. Being strong is essential for establishing your leadership within the home. With a strong leader, your kids develop a sense of safety and comfort, with the confidence they can explore their worlds. A note of caution; parents must intervene and exert their authority when life or death issues are involved. Children do not practice riding their bikes in busy streets. Adolescents do not learn by natural consequences of drugs or unsafe driving.

I have heard parents say that they think their children are smarter than they are, which justifies them giving in to their children's demands. These parents quickly develop doubt, anger and helplessness about being effective parents of such smart children. Sometimes children do have quicker minds and are intellectually more able than their parents, but parents still have the experience, the perspective and the wisdom of their years to make decisions. If you have questions about your own judgement, again, enlist the help of a person you trust. Your perspective is essential in the decision-making process. If you doubt your ability to make decisions at appropriate times, your kids are in serious trouble. Be careful about getting so caught up with how smart and wonderful your children are that you forget that you are the one who sets the standards and provides the choices on issues.

"You know, I gave Mary a choice of apple juice or milk, but she saw right through that and wanted Coke. What could I do?"

"He just talked me right out of what I thought was right. I thought I could be strong and stick to my guns, but before I knew it, I gave in and he spent the night with Jim."

"As soon as we started talking about getting up in the morning, she convinced me that she can't do it without me. What she said made sense so I wake her up and we keep getting into arguments."

Control battles as your kids near age eighteen are meaningless. By then you hope to have a relationship where you can discuss opinions and provide input as they make healthy decisions.

Many parents come to my office wanting to know

how they can get their kids to eat healthy meals, get to sleep on time, study more effectively, or simply talk to them. I remind parents that the only behavior they can control is their own, and that these problem behaviors are entirely in the child's control. Instead of asking, what can I do to change his or her behavior, ask yourself: what can I do when Johnny does not eat well, when Mary refuses to go to sleep, when Becky won't answer me, when Martha refuses to learn, when Bobby continues to soil his pants? The answers to these questions involve the parents' behavior around the issue, not getting the child to change. If in fact these problem behaviors are health-related, i.e., eating disorders, encopresis, mutism, sleep or learning disorders, you must seek professional help. If your child continues with problems, decide whether he "can't" or "won't" perform as expected.

As a parent, you know your child better than anyone. Follow your instincts and have a professional evaluation if you have concerns. If you find yours is a child who "won't," trying to force the behavior isn't going to work anyway. If your child is one who "can't," then appropriate professional intervention is necessary.

Control battles often occur around "respect." Respect battles often take place around the way kids talk to their parents.

"Don't talk to me that way. I'm your father/ mother!!"

"How can you think or say such a thing. That is not what we believe in this family."

Rudeness, foul language, disregarding the rights of others either verbally or physically are not acceptable behaviors from our children or from anyone else. It is easier for your children to follow these rules if the parents also follow them. However, even if you have trouble with your own respectfulness, you can still ask your children to comply with the standards you want within your home.

Sometimes parents think that kids are being disrespectful when they don't agree with the parents' opinions. Sometimes kids don't realize that they can disagree with us but are still expected to do what we ask.

"Please clean your room."

"I shouldn't have to clean my room."

"I know you don't think you have to, but I am requesting that you do it anyway. We have a difference of opinion about this that we can talk about later."

If you, as a parent, have no room for disagreement on any subject, be prepared to have a limited and stormy relationship with your kids. In a reciprocal, respectful relationship, kids learn there are some issues that are particularly important to you that they cannot challenge. Our children disagreed with us about the safety of motorcycles and our refusal to support their desire to purchase one. This was an area of no compromise for us, as parents.

You also learn to accept that people, including your children, hold opinions that differ from yours. A good example is curfew. Mom and Martha do not have to agree on what time is appropriate for a fifteen-year-old. They can agree to disagree about a reasonable time. But, once a curfew is established, Martha is expected to follow the house rule, even if she does not agree that it is suitable. I do not have to agree with the tax laws in order to comply with them. Once parents and kids realize how this applies in their homes, a lot of problems about respect evaporate.

Sometimes disagreements occur around issues that are within your child's complete ownership. A sixteen-year-old may decide to wear his hair in a way that you can't tolerate. You may disagree with the choice but because of his age, you realize that the hairstyle is really his decision. In this case, your child may ask you to love him by supporting him even as you disagree with each other. An eight-year-old may want to wear a favorite pair of jeans to school, but you may think they are too worn. Generally, an eight-year-old can make pretty good choices about clothes, so the problem of what to wear is really his own. Even if you disagree with his choice, let it go, and show support for your child's knowledge of what's right for him. Save your energy for issues that really make a difference.

2. The person who owns the problem is the one best suited to solve the problem.

In order for children to become adults who take care of themselves and stay safe, they must internalize a voice that says "be self-caring." The self-caring voice becomes part of them as they gain experience in making decisions and living with the consequences of their decisions. Intellectual development is important, but is not sufficient for the self-caring voice to develop. Talking about it, or telling them how consequences will feel is not enough to internalize the learning; they must have experience. In simple terms, the process goes something like this: If I do X, then Y will happen. When Y happens I feel bad. Yikes! I don't like to feel bad, so next time I think I will try Z.

Each time you do something for your children that they can do for themselves, they lose an opportunity to learn about pain or pleasure resulting from their choices. You might question how they can learn from experience when they are just babies. But remember, if your new puppy can learn where to sleep, when food is served and what to accomplish on his walk, surely your children can learn as well. They learn gradually and they learn through experience. We do not let kids discover how to budget money for the first time when they are fourteen by giving them a year's worth of allowance all at once. But they can find out at age eight that if they spend all of their allowance on candy, they won't have enough to buy a Barbie or a G.I. Joe. We don't allow kids the use of a car if they haven't already learned that when they behave recklessly they can get hurt.

In order to decide how the person who owns the problem solves it, you must know what problems are your children's to own at various ages. Then you can help them develop the skills to solve problems on their own.

For example, at age six, in first grade, most children are able and eager to select what they wear to school. Most will do this if given the chance. Problems occur when mother or father does not think the clothes are good enough or matched well and insist that the kids "look" a certain way. Another problem occurs when there is not enough time to let them dress themselves, so we do it for them, which keeps them from learning an age-appropriate task.

By age fourteen many kids are eager to manage their own money, have a checkbook, a savings account, or cook a meal. There is no reason to expect them to do any of these tasks well without instruction and guidance. Set them up for success by supporting them through the learning process rather than saying, "Oh, you think you're so smart, good luck!"

Learning how to make decisions is part of the apprenticeship program your children are involved in, with you serving as their supervisor. They have a much better chance of success if they first master small segments of larger skills. When they show an interest in mastering skills, assist them in an age-appropriate way. If a six-year-old wants to make dinner, you won't let him loose at the stove, but a six-year-old *can* learn to measure and pour and mix. A six-year-old can set the table and clear the dishes. Six-year-olds know what they like to eat and can recommend menu items.

Another problem arises when a parent expects the child to know how to perform a task without first being shown the way the parent expects it to be done. For example, there are many ways of getting dressed. Some families like to wear matching socks and shirts or have the shirt tucked in. If it is important to you that they learn to do something a particular way, spend time with your children instructing them. If you were to ask four of your friends what it means to clean a room, you would probably get four different answers. Let your children know what you want from them and then spend time with them until the task is mastered. If you want them to learn something new, guide them, teach them, take the time to do it together. Time spent at the beginning reaps huge dividends. Mastering a new skill is a four-step process:

1. Being aware of the skill, such as learning to drive, getting dressed, cleaning a room, washing clothes, cooking meals, budgeting, being a friend, cutting the lawn, taking out the trash.

2. Practicing with someone as you learn the details. Examples are Driver's Ed, getting dressed with parents, making the bed together, learning to sort the clothes, etc.

3. Performing the task with guidance and some super-

vision. Examples of this are: obtaining a learner's permit, checking with your parents about how you did, parents doing part of the room or checking in at intervals, etc.

4. Doing it on your own. Such as: getting a driver's license, shopping by yourself, cleaning the kitchen.

Still another problem develops when parents allow children to make decisions about issues that are not theirs to own. This is where we as parents can protect our children's childhood. It is no secret today that many children are forced into adult roles before they are ready. Young children come home from school to empty houses, sometimes expected to care for their brothers and sisters. One radio host told me about his afternoon program that children call into. He is serving an important role, since he is supporting many children doing homework or chores while parents work. Parents are proud of their children when they are precocious, and sometimes children are forced to perform when they are much too young. We wonder why kids are anxious to have children, buy expensive cars, drink, use drugs. One possible answer is that there is nothing left for their adolescence because that was used up when they were still children.

A tragic event occurred when seven-year-old Jessica DuBroff died in an airplane crash while attempting to become the youngest person to fly across the United States. When she took off in bad weather on the second leg of the trip from Cheyenne, Wyoming, the plane crashed and all aboard were killed. Many were flabbergasted when Jessica's mother responded with pride that her daughter died doing something she loved to do. Whether this tragedy should have happened can be debated for a long time. But here is a situation when a child was put in the position of making decisions that clearly belonged to an adult. Jessica was only seven years old and could not have had the physical or intellectual wisdom to make a wise choice about flying. She knew she liked to fly, but that is different from being the pilot. In my opinion parents need to exercise judgement that protects their children from potentially life-threatening situations. I am not referring to situations where they might be hurt, like learning to ride a bike, but situations where they might be killed. Even if we do have precocious or talented children, we still need to remember that they are children and are equipped with the limited experience of childhood. It is our responsibility to give them every chance to become adults.

Letting the person own and solve his part of the problem has major implications for parents' stress-filled lives. Most of you can easily reduce your stress and have more time for yourselves and with your families if you solve only the problems you own and provide guidance, as necessary, for the rest. Be prepared for new complaints that may arise from the person who suddenly finds himself with new responsibilities. A frequent comment when you stop solving someone else's problems is, "What's the matter, don't you love me anymore?" The answer is, "Of course, that's why I want you to learn to take care of yourself." "This stinks." And later (sometimes much later), "Thanks for your support and belief in me."

3. House rules should be clearly stated and, preferably, written down.

I cannot express strongly enough how important it is to have what you expect from each family member (including the parents) stated and, preferably, written down.

The written statement then becomes the law of the land, or house rules. The rules you decide on will reflect the values of the people who write them just as the Constitution is a reflection of the values of the founders of the United States. Our workplaces, communities, and country could not function if we didn't know the rules and the consequences if we don't comply.

There are many kids who complain about how much their parents nag:

"She keeps bugging me."

"As soon as one thing is done, he thinks of something else for me to do."

"I was just going to get to my chores, but before I could she started nagging me about the trash. Have you taken the trash out yet? What about your room? Then she called Dad into the argument."

"The only thing they care about is if I get my chores done. After I hear that voice I just don't want to do anything. I want it to be my idea but before I can get to doing the chores they're at me again. What a pain."

And then I hear:

"I have to ask him about ten times before he responds, and then he does half the job and complains that I didn't tell him what I meant."

"She never listens. She's not motivated. What am I going to do? I hate being a nag but if I don't nag, nothing gets done."

"I know I told him to go to his room for a month. Of course I didn't mean it. I was just so mad I didn't know what else to say. When he ignores me I get furious. I just don't know how I can win. Everything is against me."

At some point you must decide what you expect from your kids daily and weekly; essentially, their "job description." Imagine yourself at work without a job description. You would show up every day and then decide what your supervisor wanted you to do. You'd get paid if you guessed correctly, and did a good enough job to satisfy the supervisor. You probably wouldn't keep the job very long. Realistically, many of our kids are in this very situation. They are expected to know what we want, how we want it and when we want it. When they make a mistake, they don't know just what the consequences will be because it depends on the mood of the boss. What I usually hear from parents is, "I've told him enough times, he should know by now what I expect." That may be so, but you sure can eliminate a lot of conflict if you take the time to write down the house rules.

If you use the model of techniques that work at your job and implement it at home with your children, most problems will be solved because most kids want peace around the house as much as you do. Of course, you can't fire your kids, but they don't have much in the way of options either. Somewhere around fourteen to sixteen, kids realize that they will soon be on their own, and, therefore, don't have to put up with some of the regulations. If they feel over-regulated they often tune out, choosing to tolerate their parents' frustration and anger for a few more years until they are on their own.

You can set reasonable house rules by determining where the kids are on the Parent/Kid Triangles. Keep in mind that you want to start wherever they can experience success, even if that is far below where you believe they should be. Also, be aware of how much time you can spend with them so they can be really well trained for their jobs. Although it may be quicker to develop the job descriptions and house rules on your own, you will get much more cooperation if you involve the whole family in the decisions. If you actually assign your children the task of creating these job descriptions as well as the rewards and negative consequences, they will probably do pretty well. Most kids respond to both the challenge and the confidence you demonstrate by involving them in solving problems. Because you want to encourage each person's commitment to the rules, it is important for all parties to sign and date the contract.

There are many ways to write the rules, but the simpler the better. Include each person in the family from the baby to the parents. For instance, the baby's job might be making funny faces. Include basic rules of courtesy such as good manners, no yelling, as well as the chores. Determine the rewards for compliance and determine consequences for poor performance. Go heavy on the reward side. Rewards don't necessarily have to be money. Instead, be creative. Suggest spending extra time together or reading a favorite book. This might not suit the older kids, but you get the idea. Make copies of the house rules for each person and then post them in a conspicuous place (usually the refrigerator and/or bedroom doors) so everyone can refer to what he is expected to do. Having consequences clearly written eliminates your role as the "bad guy" because now your children can just check the sheet and know the consequences, because they helped determine them in the first place. If a new problem comes up that hasn't been covered by one of the house rules, formulate a response and then bring it up at the next family meeting.

As you develop the negative consequences, be sure to have the "punishment fit the crime." Most parents have thought it, some parents have said it; I know of only one who followed through with "You're grounded for the rest of your life!!!" If you think of developing charts, or of having an intricate form to keep track of behavior, be sure you have the organization, patience and time to follow through. Charts never worked for me. I would get involved in something and give the stickers to the kids to fill in, and before I knew it, the calendar was filled with stickers and I couldn't figure out why nothing had changed. Day-to-day time-outs, early bedtime, extra chores, or limiting TV or computer time are some acceptable consequences that do not need an accounting system.

As you list the expectations and consequences, simplicity is important, so just include the daily and weekly routines. You will not be able to think ahead to every problem you or your kids will encounter, so update the rules regularly and be prepared for the exceptional times that you never thought would happen. Kids are creative in how they live their lives and surprise you with their behavior. We had several "our kids would never do that" experiences such as when the car was driven before the driver's license was issued, and when Halloween and the "egg incident" occurred. After these "exceptional" experiences we had our kids write to us about how they needed to handle the problem. We asked them to include:

1. What they did that was wrong.
2. Why that behavior was a problem.
3. The potential consequences of the behavior.
4. How they might avoid that behavior in the future.

We have several well-thought-out statements about issues that occurred as our kids grew up. At the very least, have your children make statements to you that can answer the above questions. I prefer writing at these times because it keeps the problem in the court of the person who owned it, it gave me time to reply to their response, and it prevented a discussion of the "incident" from turning into an angry interaction. Most importantly, because the kids are writing on their own, they have to do their own thinking. The thinking and applying language to thought helps internalize the values that will guide their future actions. Young children do surprisingly well with this. If they are not comfortable writing or writing takes too much time, have a parent or an older sibling help.

Each family differs with what they want to include in the house rules. If you have not had any rules at all, too many at first can be overwhelming and lead to discouragement. Set up each family member for success by selecting rules that can be followed.

One of the rules a family can have is to respect one another. This means no hitting, screaming, yelling, or name calling and includes both parents and kids. This means no violence, verbal or physical.

Some basic expectations a family may have are a specific time to be ready for school, what chores are to be done, what time the house closes during the week and on weekends. The word curfew is intentionally avoided, as it implies a limitation of a right. Being home at a reasonable time is respectful of everyone who is living together — and provides for a level of safety for each member of the family. Bedtime, homework time and mealtimes may be covered in the house rules. You may decide to install a calendar of events posted with each person writing in a different color. Engage your children's input because they love to feel empowered within the family and are often much more creative and willing than you think.

The house rules are a good place to indicate your policies about television, movies and access to computers. I do not think that children should watch movies that are rated higher than their age. This means that videos and cable television should be evaluated by the parents. Limiting access to television can be hard on older children because they might think they have earned the right to watch a PG-13 or an R-rated movie because they have reached the magic age. I recommend that the decision be based on the age of the youngest child and provide the same level of protection for him as you did for the older ones. That would mean no R movies in the house until the youngest reaches seventeen.

Parents can say "no" to television programs that expose children to violence or sex or unacceptable values. Parents can also determine how much time is spent with the television on. Of course, it is preferable when these decisions are made cooperatively. If there are programs that you don't like but your children want to watch you might want to take the time to watch the program together. When "The Simpsons" show was first televised, I was appalled because the characters were so stereotyped and acted in ways that were very contrary to the values I wanted my children to have. But, the characters, including bratty Bart, were so appealing that they had influence. I think that "The Simpsons" is a cartoon more suited for adults than children, but the problem is that kids were relating on the most super-ficial levels to the characters who were models for very

••

unacceptable behavior. There were many disagreements (and criticisms on my part) before I decided that I would watch the program with the kids, instead of just complaining about it. At least now there was room for discussion and the children valued my opinion more because I was better informed.

There is an increasing awareness of children's access to pornographic material through computers and the Internet. Again, spending time with your children, discussing what is right and wrong, developing strong relationships, using devices on the computers to block access are ways of influencing your children's experiences. In the future there will be attempts to legislate what is acceptable, but parents still have the final responsibility.

The point is: Know what your children are watching, what they are doing and who they are doing it with. If you have any questions about how they spend their time, spend your time with them. A picture is worth a thousand words, which is one reason why video, television and computers are so powerful. Just think of the thousands of images that children are bombarded with through these media. We cannot safeguard them from everything, but by spending time with them, by providing feedback about our values, we can moderate the effect of harmful influences until they are mature enough to make decisions on their own.

4. Family meetings are essential for smooth family operations.

Time spent together creates bonds within families. Mealtimes and worshipping as a family are traditional times to be together. With the complexity of our lives, I believe that family meetings are as important to the successful operation of a family as management meetings are to the successful operation of a business. This is the opportunity to check in with each other, plan for the following week, review what has gone well and what has not. This is an opportunity for parents and kids to address the unfinished business from the previous week and air their views in order to avert future problems. It is very helpful when parents and kids are disagreeing about chores, or spending the night at a friend's, to be able to say, "We'll talk about it at the meeting. Please be sure to bring this up."

The formality of the meeting is going to depend on the family. I have seen everything from a book of minutes for each meeting to families who play a game when the "business" is completed. Usually, a particular day and time that everyone can commit to is designated as meeting time. If you cannot find a time when everyone can be together, it may tell you something about why there are some problems going on.

Family meetings are not just for discussing problems. In fact, it is important to hold them regularly even when life is great so that the meeting isn't only for crisis management. Cooperation and trust in the process are learned even when there are only minor problems to address. If meetings only address major problems, an attitude can develop that the meetings aren't fun; therefore, why bother going?

This is the ideal place to develop house rules and modify them as needed. Keep everyone involved. A side benefit of this democratic process is that the younger children will learn from the older children's input. Family meetings are wonderful opportunities for children to learn how their parents make decisions. Kids usually see only the results of their parents' thinking — in family meetings they can gain first hand experience in how decisions are made.

Chapter 22

Skills For Immediate Action

How much of this problem do I own, anyway? Once you figure this out, the rest is easy — then parents just need to behave with grace. Deciding who owns the problem, or what part of the problem you own is easy if you look at the age of your child and decide what is reasonable to expect. If you are arguing about what your child is wearing and your child is fourteen, you are involved in a problem that really doesn't belong to you. If you are arguing about homework with a ten-year-old, it may be that both of you have some responsibility in solving the problem — theirs to complete, yours to judge whether they have the ability for what they've been asked to do. If your child is having a problem with a teacher and needs a conference but does not have the skills to approach this teacher, you may want to coach him and even accompany him until he has developed the ability to do it alone. It can be very discouraging, at any age, to suddenly find yourself with a task at hand when you know you are not qualified. Adults have major stress reactions when this happens at work. Kids have major stress reactions that seems like oppositional behavior when they are suddenly asked to do something they know they are not qualified for. We can determine what is a reasonable request, then decide if they have the skills and, if they don't, we can provide the assistance they need until they master the task. Keep the Parent/Kid Triangles available as you are making your decisions!

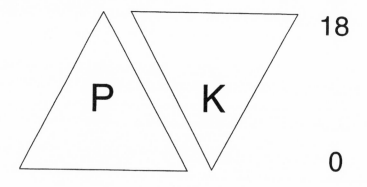

When kids reach the stage when they can and should take responsibility to get ready for school, get up on time, or stay within a budget, lots of parents say, "It's your problem; good luck." This sounds pretty unfriendly to me. Gracefully transferring the problem to the child requires sincere caring and a few kind words. In my office I use balls or stuffed animals to represent these problems. Here's how it works: During a typical conversation, the ball goes back and forth as each person tries to get the other person to keep it. If it doesn't belong to you, you toss it back with a question like, "How do you want to handle that?" or "Let me know how you work it out." You get to keep the ball if you try to come up with a solution. The last one holding the ball is the one who gets to solve the problem. When the game goes well, the rightful owner of the problem is left with the ball. If you try this with ten different balls, the balls will be spread out so that by the end of the round, no one person will have all of the responsibility. Once your hands are free of the balls that don't belong to you, you are going to have a lot more energy for yourself.

Chapter 23

Tools Of The Trade

Every coach has a set of techniques that works to get the most out of the people being coached. Coaches know that cooperation, trust and skill are the basis for winning teams. Because we are emotionally involved with our children, we sometimes let emotion influence how we get along with them. This next section contains tools for coaching that you can use with your kids so that the atmosphere stays healthy, so that you maintain your dignity and provide the best opportunity for healthy interaction.

I have printed each of the following actions on a laminated card so I can carry them around with me as reminders of the healthiest ways to approach child-rearing problems. I use cards rather than trying to remember these techniques because I need something real, not conceptual, to help me stay in a thinking state rather than falling into an emotional state. When I am challenged, or perceive that I am being challenged, I get anxious and I start reacting, usually by talking. I have finally learned and accepted how reactive I am. Sometimes I say things I regret. Once the words are out of my mouth, they can't be taken back. So I've developed external reminders of what to do in emotional circumstances.

I prefer to have more than one technique available because if I used the same method every time I would get bored and start thinking on the spot, which usually translates into reacting. I'm not a robot, and I find that I need variety or I tend to go back to the "other" ways. Also, I like to keep the other guys (the children I'm with) guessing about what I'm going to do. Kids find their parents or any adults they are around for a while very predictable and have developed set ways to respond. If they're caught off guard, then they have to think before they respond. Even though I want to get around battles, that doesn't mean that *they* do. I've learned that my best defense is good preparation. Because I am not into winning at all costs, often I just need to neutralize the effectiveness of their attack.

Remain In The Adult State. When in the adult state I can be objective, maintain my perspective and be thoughtful. I picture my actual age and my emotional age and decide to respond as the older of the two. An adult maintains self-control and has the best interests of both parties in mind. I might say something like, "That's very interesting; let me think about it, I'll get back to you," or "Thank you for letting me know." I can even ask myself how someone else might handle this. "Well, if I were Jean, what would I do?" Once I am free of the automatic hold of my emotions, more caring interaction can occur.

Eye Contact, Touch And A Smile. These are the three conditions for healthy human interaction. Ask yourself: Am I able to make eye contact? Can I smile at this person?

Would I be willing to touch him or be touched? If not, put the discussion off until a later time. If the problem is with your ability to do these things, ask why you are reacting the way you are.

A word of caution. You must be careful with touch. Who is the person you are with? Is it appropriate for you to touch him? Should you ask permission before you reach out? If this is a teenager decide whether touch is easy with him, or is he in a physically defensive, but otherwise open, stage? Does touch mean a hug or a pat on the shoulder or arm?

Voice Control. Whose voice can you control? Only your own! Listen carefully to yourself. If you ever wonder what you sound like when you're upset, place a tape recorder near the scene of frequent action. Kids often complain that parents are yelling at them and the parents claim they're not. Even if the voice is not loud, be aware of the rest of the non-verbal message. Your irritation and judgment can be stronger than the words, and kids may react as though you are yelling. Family videos and audio tapes of arguments have done more for family awareness than weeks of therapy. When talking with your children, keep your voice normal, as though you were talking with a friend. If you notice the familiar signs of increasing intensity, pitch, volume, speed, choice of words, calm yourself. Take time to breathe or leave the scene. If voice control is not possible, it's time to leave the scene, take a deep breath, and wait.

Avoid Content, Respond To The Feeling. Unless you are in a problem-solving mode or have been asked for an explanation, commenting on your kids' conversation can be perceived as a lecture and lead to an argument. For example, Brian comes home complaining about the teacher (friend, coach): "She's so mean. I can't stand her; that teacher of mine is a pain in the neck". You respond, "She was probably just having a bad day. She's one of the nicest people I know." "Thanks, Dad, whose side are you on anyway? I knew you wouldn't understand. Adults are all alike!" End of conversation.

However, if you respond to Brian's feeling, instead of content:

"You really are angry with her"

"I haven't heard you that upset in quite a while"

"I didn't realize this was bothering you so much."

He then responds: "Yeah, you wouldn't believe what happened — let me tell you about it."

Of course, there are no guarantees, but the chance for communication increases. Have you ever been in a situation where you have been disappointed with a grade? Compare, "I can't believe you can't do any better than that" to "That's a pretty upsetting grade," or "I'm sorry it worked out that way for you." Brian probably feels worse than you do about the grade — at least he should if ownership of the problem has been well designated. This does not mean that you don't care about how he feels about what's happened to him. You just don't respond as though it happened to you or that someone else has a better point of view.

Leave The Scene. This is a bit more difficult with a small child, but if you are sure that the child is safe for five minutes (or even fifteen seconds), a change of scenery can often do you a lot of good. Once out of the fire, thinking can occur. "I'll be right back" is a short phrase that can save you.

. . . .

Leave the scene is a time-out for parents — a time-out to breathe and to think about what to do. Buy some time. When you leave the scene, be careful that you are not implying that you are abandoning the child. I have seen kids who are frantic when their parents leave the room because they have had experience with parents leaving and not returning for extended periods of time. If you are worried that your child gets so angry that he will burn the house down or hurt himself or be otherwise destructive if you leave, I recommend that you seek professional help.

There are also times when it's necessary for the kids to leave the scene — these are time-outs for kids. This is not banishment. Time-outs can be effective when your child knows that he can return to the normal family activities when he is able to appropriately follow the house rules. Time-outs are not groundings or punishments designed to hurt them. Instead, the time-out is an opportunity to get back self-control.

Coach. Remember that it's often best to coach rather than parent. If you act as a coach, then there are no lectures and the resulting ill-will. You decide your next step rather than rehashing the past, and ultimately you realize you are both on the same team. When you think of yourself as your kid's coach rather than parent, you are more likely to concentrate on how he can use his strengths rather than on what limits his success. Your intention is for both of you to win.

Change The Pace. Whatever the pace of the conversation, change it. If your speech is fast and anxious, slow it down, pausing between words. Whatever you do, speak with intent. Get out of automatic. If you are speaking slowly and deliberately, speak with a quieter tone. Notice your pace, change it. Notice the pace of the child's speech pattern and switch to a different mode. Intentional action rather than automatic reaction is the goal.

Broken Record. This is particularly effective when you have made a request that your child is attempting to avoid by giving all the good reasons it shouldn't be done. This technique is easy. Firmly and quietly, restate your request.

"It's time to take the dog out."

"But Mom."

"It's time to take the dog out."

"But Mom, this program just started and I...."

"It's time to take the dog out."

"But Mom, that's not fair, you're always picking on me."

"It's time to take the dog out" (the voice stays cool).

"Gees, Mom, what's wrong with you? You sure have gotten weird lately."

You can probably have a lot of fun with this by sounding like an android: "It's time — to take — the dog — out!" or, "It's time, it's time." This can also work with changing the pace. Catch them off guard, use humor. This can be fun — for both of you.

Agree With What You Hear. No one can argue alone. When kids want to argue, they can aggravate you into a negative response and use that negative energy to their advantage as they develop a strong offense. What a surprise it is if you go with *their* energy and agree.

"Everybody else's dad is letting them go. You're

such a nerd."

Answer, "You may be right," instead of, "Don't call me that."

"Dad this is the worst day of my life."

Answer, "I'm sorry it's so bad," instead of, "There you go again with that negative attitude."

"Mom, you're so weird."

Answer, "Thank you for noticing," instead of, "How dare you say that to me."

"I know I can't get this done."

Answer, "You may not," instead of, "Don't give up, keep on trying, I know you can do it."

I Feel, When, Because. The statement, "I feel _____ when _____ because _____" belongs on the refrigerator right next to the Parent/Kid Triangles and the list of house rules. This statement is necessary for honest, intimate disclosure, which is the basis of communication. When families come in for counseling claiming they have a problem communicating, it is often because they are busy noticing and criticizing each other. The complainers are usually interested in changing someone else and believe that if only the other person would change, everything would be okay. By using this statement there is an opportunity for self reflection and disclosure.

However, this statement can be misused because so many people use it to freely express their opinions rather than their feelings. Here's an example:

"My therapist told me that it's okay and important for me to tell you how I feel. Are you ready? Here goes — I feel that you never pay attention to me. I feel that you don't love me anymore. I feel that you act like the biggest jerk that I've ever met."'

Wrong! This is probably not what your therapist had in mind — at least I hope not.

Compare that interaction to this:

"I feel worried when I don't get attention from you because I think you don't love me anymore."

"I feel embarrassed when I am with you and you act like that because I don't want people to think I made a mistake when I married you."

If the words "like" or "that" are used after the word "feel," the statement changes from an expression of emotion to an expression of opinion. You can always argue with an opinion, because there are so many opinions and points of view. You cannot argue with feelings; you feel how you feel. Please notice how you use this phrase. Once you become aware of the distinction between expressing your opinions and your feelings you will be able to start communicating much more effectively.

Stop, Breathe, Think, Respond. When you notice your cues of increasing emotion such as a loud voice, talking fast, clenched fists, hot face, tears starting, an upset stomach or cursing, *stop,* take a moment to *breathe* a deep, cleansing, relaxing breath (out and in). Take as many breaths as you need to become focused. *Think* about what you are going to do or say, then *respond* by taking whatever action you decide. You may decide to respond by doing nothing. Unless there is a life-threatening situation, there is no need to resolve a problem at the moment it occurs.

Concentrate On The Goal. When you keep in mind the purpose for the conversation, you stay focused on the route you have to take to get there — you can't be talked into taking a side trip. In Arlington, Texas, this is referred to as taking a trip to Dallas, and before you know it you find yourself heading to Waco. The dialogue goes something like this:

"But everyone is going, Mom."

"I understand dear, and I realize how upset you are."

"I really want to go."

"I understand that, dear."

"Get out of the dark ages. You never let me do anything."

"Of course I do. Just last week you went and spent the day with Brad," etc.

When you concentrate on the goal, you can ignore the tone of someone's voice and the words that are used. Instead, you address these problems later in a family meeting or a planned opportunity to clear the air after the heat has dissipated. Does this mean you sometimes let your children have the last word? Yes. This is not giving in, since the issue is addressed at a later time.

You do not have to defend your decisions to your children although you may want them to understand how you reached your conclusion. Explaining is a reasonable thing to do if they really want to know the reason. But beware; kids are usually more interested in getting you to change your mind.

When your child is questioning why they can't spend the weekend with a friend, respond only if the request is made to help your child understand the reasons for your decision. I caution parents about answering questions when the information they provide is then used to argue. If you find yourself defending your decisions, stop the conversation and let them know that you will continue when they can listen, not argue.

Sidestep Control Battles. In sidestepping a control battle, offer options whenever possible. Be sure these choices are things you can live with and that you can follow through with if necessary. Do only what you have to do and leave the rest of the problem solving to the kid. Address the problem that was at the root of the conflict at a later time, or you will probably see it surface again.

Good Neighbor Policy. This is simple enough: Respond to your child the same way you would respond to a friend, or someone you want to see again. Now you might not get a friendly response from your child initially, but this is not a case of "an eye for an eye." Because it's "not fair" that you are nice and they are not, shouldn't cause you to sink to their level. Being a better parent is about doing the "right" thing even when it is tough.

There are times that you may think that your child is not a person you would choose to spend any time with, so, why treat him like a friend? It may end up that you will not have a close relationship when they grow up, but for now, you are the adult; at least, be proud of *your* behavior.

Chapter 24

Planning Ahead – Speaker/Listener Technique

The speaker/listener technique is a concrete way of interacting not just talking but really communicating. When one person speaks and the other is listening, a message that is sent has a chance of being heard and understood. In this case, listening does not mean problem solving or changing behavior — it means simply acknowledging what is said. The technique presented here is a modification of work for couples done by Howard Markman's group from the University of Denver. Although the technique was developed for adults, it works beautifully with children who often have difficulty being heard by "big people."

This is the way it works. The family has a tile that is identified as the "talking tile," a tool to be used during discussions or family meetings. The Markmans use a piece of linoleum that is referred to as "The Floor." This is surprisingly effective. Most kids laugh or groan about the tile, but they are happy to have something concrete rather than theoretical or conceptual as they talk. The tile is a reminder of their role as the speaker or listener as well.

Although I am commenting on the benefits to the children, most adults are happy about using the tile for the same reasons.

The rules are simple — The person who holds the tile is the speaker; the other person is the listener. The speaker makes statements about a particular subject. The statements are his or her opinions or feelings — they are *not* about the other person. The listener repeats to the speaker what he hears — he does not interpret or summarize — he merely repeat the words back as closely as he can. If the listener forgets what was said, he may ask the speaker to repeat. The "session" should last no longer than ten minutes. Problem-solving is done later. Here's an example: The topic for discussion is household chores:

Speaker : "I am angry that I have so much work to do. It doesn't seem fair that I have so much to do and Mary gets off so easy."

Listener: "I hear that you are angry that you have so much work to do. It doesn't seem fair that you have so much to do and Mary gets off so easy."

Speaker: "That's right. When the list was made out I wasn't there and I got stuck with the worst stuff. I think you guys were picking on me and gave me the bathroom. This always happens to me."

Listener: "I hear that when the list was made out you weren't there and you got stuck with the worst stuff. You think we were picking on you and gave you the bathroom. You think this always happens to you."

Speaker: "Yeah — what are you going to do about it?"

Listener: "I hear that you want to know what I'm

going to do about it."

At this point the speaker has decided that he has said enough, and they agree to change places. The speaker gives the tile to the listener.

New Speaker: "I didn't know you were so upset about the chores. Thanks for telling me. I think you expressed yourself very well."

Listener: "You said that you didn't know I was so upset about the chores. You thanked me for telling you. You think I expressed myself very well."

Speaker: "Just as a reminder, we are not going to do any problem-solving just now. Let's talk about it tomorrow night."

Listener: "You said that just as a reminder, we are not going to do any problem-solving just now. You want to talk about it tomorrow night."

Doesn't this sound ideal? What is so surprising is how well kids do when they are not being confronted, criticized or otherwise feeling attacked and backed into a corner. It's also amazing how well parents can speak when they are not being challenged, criticized, verbally attacked or think they have to defend their decisions. Parents are very impressed with how well children respond when the conversation has been equalized by the small tile. Children as young as four years old have been able to use this surprisingly well. The "talking tile," or "floor," is placed in an accessible spot at home. The most frequent initial complaint from parents or adults is that they think that don't need something as elementary as this to "really communicate." These complaints quickly dissipate once they experience the effects of a real conversation with their kids.

Here's another example:

Speaker: "I feel sad when no one is home for dinner because it's so lonely for me."

Listener: (immediate first reaction when defending) "I had to work late. There was no one there to take my place. I knew this job wasn't going to work out well. Oh, they'll never forgive me. Boy, all you do is complain. Where do they think I get the money for those expensive shoes? Well, you haven't been home for dinner on time for the last three years — don't get so huffy with me."

It's very hard to listen to the message when you're so busy defending yourself or justifying your own behavior. Try this, instead:

Listener: "I hear that you feel sad when no one is home for dinner because it's so lonely for you."

One value in this technique is the listener is so busy listening to the words he doesn't have time to be defensive or critical. Most people I have worked with have found that they lose track of what is said when they start thinking about defending themselves.

If you are the listener and can't remember what has been said because it was confusing or was too long to remember, just say so and ask for the speaker to repeat. But stay with the exercise until you get it right. Ideally, the speaker should use short sentences, and only a few at a time, to make it easier for the listener to hear.

This technique is especially effective with topics that are highly emotional. Often emotion is expressed as anger, with a loud voice and hostile words. Anger is usually a secondary emotion coming from deeper feelings of sadness or fear. When there is lots of emotion — and the emotion you usually need protection from is anger — simply make one statement or sentence and then have the listener repeat it. As elementary as this sounds, it works. If the emotion, such as anger, is still too volatile for either party to feel safe, then the topic is tabled to be addressed again within 24 hours. Again, if you have tried everything and it still doesn't work, seek professional help.

The rules again:

1. The topic to be discussed is decided on before you begin.
2. The speaker holds the tile and makes statements about his own feelings and opinions. Avoid name-calling, labeling or mind reading. Statements made are strictly related to the topic.
3. The listener reiterates to the speaker what has just been said. The listener responds when asked to by the speaker, when he asks permission to respond or after each statement.
4. When the speaker is ready to relinquish the tile, the speaker and listener roles are exchanged with the new speaker now making statements relevant to the issue and the new listener repeating what is said.
5. This is a time for communicating — *not* problem-solving. Problem-solving, if necessary, is accomplished within 24 hours.

Using the speaker/listener technique with the tile is not a complicated process and can be quite enlightening. In a family therapy session, a woman has brought her husband into counseling complaining about a lack of communication:

"He never listens."

Husband says, "I do so listen."

"No, you don't."

"Yes, I do."

The conversation continues with each one telling the other one what he/she does wrong and with he/she defending his/her behavior. I summarize what I've heard, get agreement from the couple and suggest we try something. Once I have permission, out comes the tile. The husband speaks first as his wife is coached to listen. Within a few minutes, she is repeating back as the listener. Now the roles are switched, and she speaks. Then he responds, is coached, tries again and is amazed with the difficulty he had repeating what his wife has said. He is an intelligent, successful person. Why the difficulty? He has been trained to get to the heart of the matter, to summarize, to interpret, to be a man of action. He is also hesitant about coming into "therapy," since this is his wife's idea. He has to replace the cruise control of his communication style with a standard shift. Once this exercise was completed, he was agreeable and understanding of what his wife's complaints were about his not listening. They both had a sense of satisfaction because by his listening more, she felt increasingly valued.

Chapter 25

Create A Great Place To Live

A warm environment that supports open communication and safety is important for responsible, healthy living. Within the frantic day there must be a time for peace, to recuperate from stress. Let your home be a place of emotional and physical safety. After basic needs are met, further development can occur.

Now, take a moment to imagine that you are walking in the front door of your home. Look around and notice what is there. Begin walking through your home, taking the time to enter each room. Become aware of what you learn about the people who live here. You are probably pretty satisfied with what you experience. Now, how can you make your home *great*?

Increasing evidence indicates that what we experience through our senses affects the way we think, feel and behave. Retail shops use aromas to encourage customers to buy more. Some prisons are experimenting with aromas to calm the prisoners. Remember the smell of Christmas and how relaxing certain aromas are. Colors also affect our moods. There is a definite difference between being in a red room or a yellow one. Having a neat home can certainly lower stress if you know where to look for things, since clutter and chaos can cause confusion.

I was pleased with a report from a teacher who had attended one of my workshops introducing the idea of using aromas for affecting moods. She had a Thanksgiving project for her class that involved cooking apples with cloves and cinnamon. While cooking she decided to overdo it on the spices, and the sweet smells permeated the room. She reported that within a few minutes the kids were talking about warm holiday memories — mostly about their grandmothers who did a lot of cooking, especially apple pie. Although this would not qualify as a controlled experiment, she was certainly impressed by the results.

Advertisers have studied psychology and know how to affect your decisions. You can take a page from their book and use it in your own home to create a place that is soothing and pleasant and reflects the people who live there. You can even let your kids participate in choosing certain colors in their rooms and in places they like to spend time. Their choices may not always reflect your taste, but you might find that by cooperating and including them in the decisions, their sense of ownership will also increase their sense of pride. Help your children keep their rooms and their personal space neat. This may seem like an impossible request but the task becomes easier when anything your children cannot care for by themselves is eliminated from their rooms. Many parents have been shocked by this suggestion because they spent so much money on toys and other gifts. Most kids have much more than they need, they often have everything they want. If their "stuff" and taking care of it is causing problems, reduce the "stuff" and you might also reduce the problems.

You do not have to spend a lot of money to change the atmosphere in the house. Most homes have radios; turn the station to one that plays music. Turn off the television. Boil some water on the stove and put in some cinnamon and cloves and apple slices. Use candles to soften the lighting. Turn an old piece of cloth into a table scarf. Experiment. This is your home; find something that works for you.

Recently, a young mother with four children under seven came in to see me. After a recent move and being in temporary quarters, the family organization was all but gone, and the stress was extremely high. (Not surprisingly.) Playtime, mealtime, bath and bedtime were all difficult. As we did some problem-solving it became apparent that the parents were going to need some assistance in effecting change. Unfortunately, due to the recent move there was no extended family available, and the new social support system (neighborhood, school and church) was not yet in place. Several suggestions were made for what could be done within the home, which included a daily schedule and finding tapes with relaxation music and using aromas in the house to help with a general state of relaxation. These were also recommended to be used at bath time, which was right before bedtime. There are several bath oils that will not dry out your children's skin (but if you have any questions, talk to your primary care physician) and that are made with essential oils. A selection of these, such as lavender or hops, can assist the calming of the body, mind and spirit. Not only will your children become calmer, you will, too. Having particular music that is used just at bath and bedtime will soon be associated with winding down and the end of the day. As you towel them dry, you may wish to massage them, which will also calm them.

Regarding music: There are often very strong differences of opinion between what kids like and what parents like. Don't impose your taste on everyone else, but do set a standard that is comfortable for you. If your older teenagers have CDs that are distasteful to you, ask them to play them outside of the house. You may decide to remove offensive music from younger children completely. They may listen to that music someplace else; you certainly have no control over that, but you can make a statement as to your values.

The importance of meals, and especially meals together as a family, cannot be overlooked. Turn off the TV, sit down together, eat at the same time. It does not matter what you serve, but it does matter that you eat together. There needs to be a time to connect daily and I think mealtime is that time. It is not just coincidence that many religious ceremonies involve sharing of bread and water or wine or a meal. Make this a sacred time and let the meal become not just food for the body, but for the family.

I have wonderful memories of returning home to the delicious smells of food filling the house. My mother cooked every day. On Saturdays there were yeasty smells of fresh rolls. Each Saturday morning the baking was done. Sugar, yeast, chicken, pot roast, garlic, onion, tomatoes, cinnamon infused the warm, humid kitchen and warmed our hearts. How rich the scents and the memories evoked even as I write these words. I wonder what this generation of children will relate to? The ring of the pizza delivery service and the red-and-blue Domino's box? MTV? The house just doesn't smell the same when the pizza is delivered to the front door, compared to the sauce simmering on the stove and the garlic browning in the oven. The scents, sounds, sights, and memories are what bind us to the generations before us. Ritual and tradition are important in grounding us and providing us with a sense of place and time, reference points in this journey called life.

Because many of us no longer have our extended families to support us, the job of raising our children is often something we are doing alone. Raising children is work and can be exhausting. Instead of being able to send them to Grandma's or Grandpa's for the afternoon where they could spend time with people who love them and whose values are close to our own, we often send them to the TV or the radio or the music or the movies where they receive information which can affect their values. Therein lies a big danger that we must be aware of if we want our children to incorporate our values into their system. If you do not have family around to support you and help raise the next generation, take the time to seek out people of like values and beliefs. This often happens within religious communities. Build and become part of a community that serves as a surrogate family if you do not have one around. A note of caution: Do not think that just because you share religious beliefs or family ties that you share values. While this might be true, be cautious with the people you choose to have your children spend time with. Try to connect in your community with people who have similar values, and get to know them before you assume that your children will be safe with them. It takes time but can be worth it ultimately.

The most important ingredient for a great environment is time. Attention to how your home looks, smells or sounds is the beginning of making a great place to live. But without time for each other, each of the elements remain separate. It is the time together that works magic in a house to make it a home. Time has been praised and cursed — it flies by, drags, gets lost, wasted, sometimes found, often worried about. The bottom line is that we each get the same amount every day, and children need time with the people they love and rely on to develop attachments, relationships, values, a sense of belonging and of being loved in return. We tell our children we love them and we mean it, but it is through the choices we make that we show them what our priorities really are. Kids love being number one. Children love having their parents show up at school, watch their sports, read to them, care about homework, sit with them, play games with them, cook for them, eat with them, have bedtime together. As children become older and become more independent, parent availability and ease of access continue to be important.

With your many busy schedules, examine where you want your children to be in your time frame and, if you have to, write your time with them in on your daily planner and honor that as though it were an appointment with the President of the United States. When you find that you are required to be away from home, stay in contact with your family. Leave messages to your children about where you are, when you expect to return, and how they can contact you if they need you. If you are out of town, call on the telephone, leave notes for them to read while you are gone.

When all is said and done, the most important part of your children's environment is you. Being a better parent requires time and interest, which seem like small requirements for such great rewards.

Conclusion

Here it is: a guide for you to become better parents so you can have stronger kids. For those of you who want to make major changes, remember to give yourself the necessary time and space for change to occur. Imagine the progress you would like to see in a year, and start planning and implementing small changes today. Keep track of your successes, no matter how small, so when you become disheartened you can look back and realize your accomplishments.

Our children are gifts who will always live in our hearts even as they grow more independent. As children they rely on us for their well-being. We owe it to them to provide for their needs while treating them with dignity and acting with integrity. In our fast-paced industrialized, technologically sophisticated society that spins and skyrockets so quickly, we can easily lose our selves and our children, spiritually as well as physically. As a parent who nearly lost her child, and with that awareness realized how easy it was to lose herself, I offer this guidance and information to you with love and best wishes.

To order additional copies of

Dr. Gaffney's Coaching Guide
for
Better Parents and Stronger Kids
Book: $12.95   Shipping/Handling $3.50

or

Dr. Gaffney's Coaching Guide
for
Relaxation and Meditation

Audio tape and booklet: $14.95   Shipping /Handling $2.50

Call BookPartners, Inc.
1-800-895-7323

To contact Dr. Carol Gaffney for personal coaching,
seminars, speaking appearances, newsletter or
other educational products

Phone: 1-888-DrGaffney
or
Web page site: http://www.drgaffney.com
e-mail address: carol@drgaffney.com